privacy in the ONLINE WORLD

Online Privacy and Health Care

Melissa Abramovitz

ReferencePoint Press®

San Diego, CA

ReferencePoint Press®

About the Author

Melissa Abramovitz has been a freelance writer for more than twenty-five years and specializes in writing nonfiction magazine articles and books for all age groups. She is the author of hundreds of magazine articles, more than thirty educational books for children and teenagers, numerous poems and short stories, several children's picture books, and a book for writers.

Printed in the United States

For more information, contact:
ReferencePoint Press, Inc.
PO Box 27779
San Diego, CA 92198
www. ReferencePointPress.com

Picture Credits
Cover: Thinkstock Images; © Mario Anzuoni/Reuters/Corbis: 14; © Bettmann Corbis: 10; © Rick Gomez/Corbis: 36; © Karen Kasmauski/Corbis: 33; © Helen King/Corbis: 20; © National Geographic Society/Corbis: 17; Science Source: 29; Thinkstock Images: 25, 45, 51, 56, 61; © Leigh Vogel/Corbis: 41

LIBRARY OF CONGRESS CATALOGING-IN-PUBLICATION DATA

Abramovitz, Melissa, 1954–
Online privacy and health care / by Melissa Abramovitz.
pages cm. — (Privacy in the online world)
Audience: Grade 9 to 12.
Includes bibliographical references and index.
ISBN-13: 978-1-60152-652-6 (hardback)
ISBN-10: 1-60152-652-0 (hardback)
1. Internet in medicine—Juvenile literature. 2. Medical informatics—Security measures—Juvenile literature. 3. Health services administration—Computer network resources—Juvenile literature. I. Title.
R859.7.I58A27 2015
610.285—dc23

2013044631

Contents

Threats to Health Care Privacy

In July 2013 Cedars Sinai Hospital in Los Angeles fired six workers for illegally looking at the electronic hospital records of fourteen patients. Four of the workers were employed by doctors who treated patients at the hospital. One was a hospital medical assistant, and one was a student research assistant. All used passwords they should not have had access to. Five of the six accessed the records of only one patient—actress Kim Kardashian, after Kardashian gave birth to her daughter North West.

None of the workers had any legitimate reason to look at patient files. In doing so, they violated hospital policies and federal Health Insurance Portability and Accountability Act (HIPAA) laws. HIPAA rules are the main federal laws that govern patient privacy in the United States. Despite these rules, however, many hospital employees snoop in electronic patient records out of curiosity or to sell the information. This happens everywhere. It has, however, been especially prevalent in Los Angeles, where many celebrities such as Kardashian live.

The Lure of Snooping

The University of California–Los Angeles (UCLA) hospitals have had even more problems with employee snooping than other area hospitals. Many of the UCLA file breaches were traced to administrative specialist Lawanda Jackson. Jackson began using her supervisor's password to access patient files in 2004. Her main targets were celebrity patients such as pop star Britney Spears, actress Farrah Fawcett, and former California first lady Maria Shriver. Unlike many hospital employees who violate patient privacy laws out of simple curiosity, Jackson broke additional laws when she sold celebrity patient information to the *National Enquirer*.

Jackson was caught after Fawcett set up a "sting" operation. Fawcett was upset about frequent *National Enquirer* reports about her medical consultations at UCLA. She suspected that the tabloid was getting information from someone at the hospital and intended to prove it. She and her doctor told no one, including family members, that her cancer had returned. After the *Enquirer* reported that Fawcett's cancer was back, UCLA began an investigation which led them to Lawanda Jackson's computer.

Jackson initially told the *Los Angeles Times* that "it was just me being nosy. . . . It wasn't for money or anything."[1] Evidence that the *National Enquirer* deposited $4,600 in her husband's checking account after the Fawcett story was published, however, proved otherwise. Further evidence showed that Jackson inappropriately accessed 939 patient files. She resigned before she could be fired in 2007 and later pleaded guilty in court to charges of violating HIPAA laws for financial gain. Jackson's punishment for these transgressions would have been fines of up to $250,000, plus up to ten years in prison, but she died of cancer before the sentence could be imposed.

Lawanda Jackson was not the only UCLA hospital employee who accessed medical files for no legitimate reason. In fact, the federal government's Department of Health and Human Services Office for Civil Rights (OCR) began an investigation of three hospitals in the UCLA Health System in 2009 for repeated HIPAA violations. The violations continued even after UCLA received several warnings and was fined by the state of California. OCR launched their investigation after California fined UCLA $95,000 for privacy breaches involving singer Michael Jackson, whose body was taken there after he died from a drug overdose. The investigation revealed that the privacy rights of 1,041 celebrity and noncelebrity patients were violated between 2005 and 2009. The federal government imposed a fine of $865,500 and required that UCLA hospitals retrain all their employees and enhance their computer security.

The Importance of Patient Privacy

The punishments for violating patient privacy are severe because the US government and its citizens believe that health care privacy is

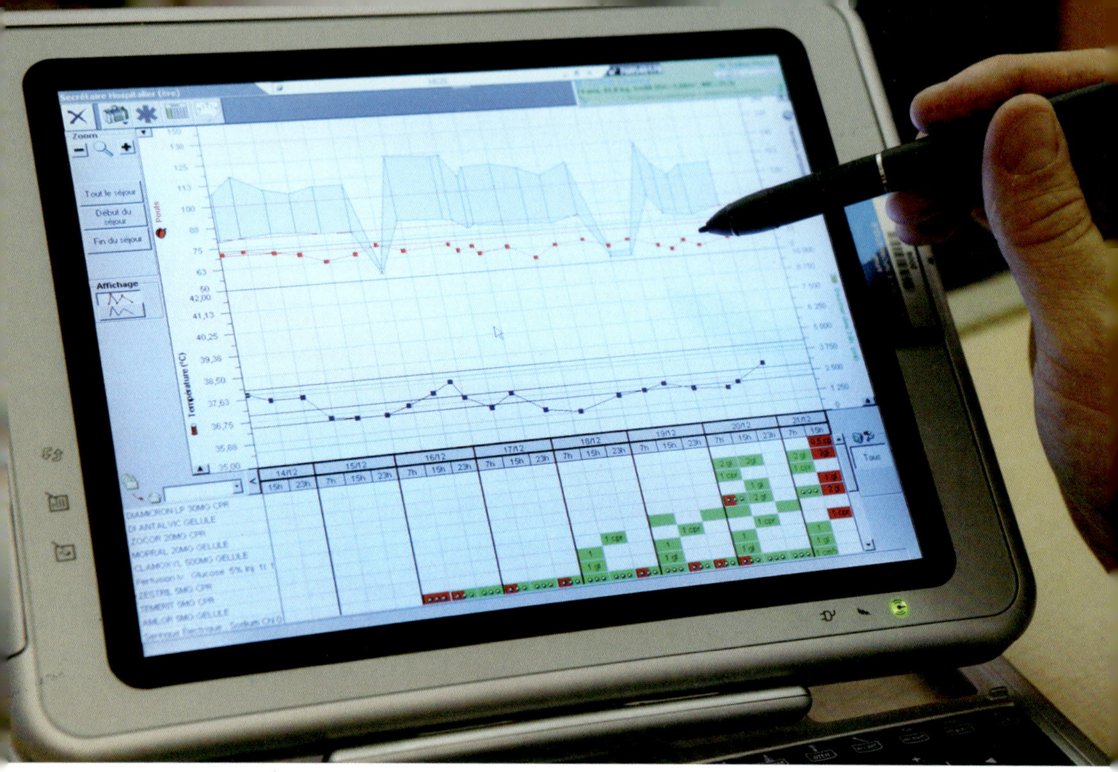

Electronic medical records (pictured) enable doctors, nurses, and other specialists to access a patient's health history and monitor ongoing treatment, both of which are essential to providing quality care. But patient privacy is threatened by online breaches.

important. People value their privacy in other areas of life as well. However, since medical records contain intimate details about individuals' mental and physical health, medical privacy is regarded as being especially important.

When doctors and hospitals treat patients, they are required by medical ethics and by law to keep information about them confidential. Confidentiality is important for several reasons. According to an Institute of Medicine and National Research Council publication, "Without some assurance of privacy, people may be reluctant to provide candid and complete disclosures of sensitive information even to their physicians."[2] In some cases, people whose medical information is breached stop seeking medical care at all. Disclosures of sensitive information can also have consequences such as broken relationships, loss of employment, loss of insurance, embarrassment, stigmatization, and identity theft. Some of these consequences result from the fact that medical records contain details such as Social Security numbers and insurance information.

Guarding Against Privacy Breaches

Protecting medical privacy, however, has become increasingly difficult in the online world, as more and more medical records are kept in electronic databases. Some of these databases are readily accessible online. Others are breached by hackers. People steal or inappropriately access health data for a variety of reasons, including curiosity, financial gain, leverage in legal cases, and retaliation. One hacker who downloaded medical and financial data on five thousand patients at the University of Washington Medical Center did so just to prove how vulnerable electronic records are.

OCR estimates that nearly 23 million people's health information has been improperly accessed in the United States since breach reporting started in 2009. A 2012 report on cybersecurity confirms that computer security in the health care field is indeed very weak. As computer security expert Avi Rubin of Johns Hopkins University states in a *Washington Post* article, "I have never seen an industry with more gaping security holes."[3] Rubin points out that health care workers tend to be lax about protecting passwords and that hospital computer systems are not guarded by strong firewalls and other protections. Computer security programs are also not updated as often as they should be.

> "I have never seen an industry with more gaping security holes."[3]
>
> —*Computer security expert Avi Rubin.*

Unauthorized breaches also occur because medical records compiled by one doctor are available to other doctors within a health network. The files are also shared with the government for research and other purposes. Under the new Affordable Care Act, these files will be shared with even more government departments in the new Federal Data Services Hub. According to Diane Black and Patrick Meehan of the US House of Representatives, "The data hub is a prime target for identity thieves and cyber attacks, and it requires the strongest possible security measures to prevent breaches."[4]

Staying a step ahead of hackers and others who abuse computer technology is increasingly challenging in all aspects of life in the twenty-first century. However, given the unique nature of medical care, the threats to health care privacy are especially serious.

Chapter 1

The Importance of Privacy

Humans need and value privacy. This need has been expressed and protected in different ways in different cultures throughout history. As Clark University professor of philosophy Judith Wagner DeCew writes, "Although not all societies protect privacy in the same way, in virtually every society individuals engage in patterns of behavior and adopt avoidance rules in order to seek privacy."[5]

People in different societies value and make rules about different types of privacy that are important to them. These types include privacy of the body, territory, personal information, and communications. Each type of privacy is not equally important in all cultures. For example, when Christopher Columbus and other European explorers first came to America, they discovered that people in some Native American tribes did not wear clothes. This meant that these tribes did not value this type of bodily privacy. In some tribes several families lived together in homes that had no separate rooms, indicating that they did not value territorial privacy within their tribe. In Europe, on the other hand, many people in the sixteenth century and afterward aspired to build houses with many separate rooms to give them privacy and social status.

Defending one's country or tribe from intruders or invaders seeks to protect another type of territorial privacy—the separation of societies with physical or virtual borders described on maps. The idea of separate countries, states, cities, and neighborhoods is indeed a manifestation of peoples' need to create boundaries between themselves and others.

Social Privacy

In addition to using rooms and houses to separate individuals or family groups from others, many cultures throughout history have viewed a family's home as symbolizing the separation of private family life from social life. One of the earliest written references to social privacy, which is a subtype of territorial privacy, appears in the book *Politics*, written by the Greek philosopher Aristotle in 350 BCE. Aristotle distinguishes the public sphere of political activity from the private sphere of personal and family life. He calls the public sphere *polis* and the private sphere *oikos*. Aristotle also writes that part of a government's job is to protect the private rights of individuals while balancing those rights with the common good. This belief influenced later philosophers and political and legal scholars, and remains a major concern of modern governments.

> "Although not all societies protect privacy in the same way, in virtually every society individuals engage in patterns of behavior and adopt avoidance rules in order to seek privacy."[5]
>
> *—Clark University professor of philosophy Judith Wagner DeCew.*

Another view of privacy that had a strong effect on later views and laws is that of the seventeenth-century British philosopher and physician John Locke. In his book *The Second Treatise of Civil Government,* Locke writes that each man is born "with a title to perfect freedom" and with the power "to preserve his property, that is, his life, liberty and estate against the injuries and attempts of other men."[6] Locke also writes that the same rights that allow individuals to own and protect property give them the power to keep personal issues, information, and communications private: "Every man has a property in his own person: this no body has any right to but himself."[7]

Privacy laws throughout the world grew out of the privacy theories of Aristotle, Locke, and others who viewed privacy as a right and government protection of this right as essential. Privacy laws also encompass the fact that privacy involves the ability of individuals to control how much information about themselves may be accessed by others, including the government. Privacy laws seek to balance this control with a government's need to protect its citizens. George Washington University law professor Daniel J. Solove explains, "Privacy is both a positive and a negative right; it is not just a freedom from the state, but also a duty of the state

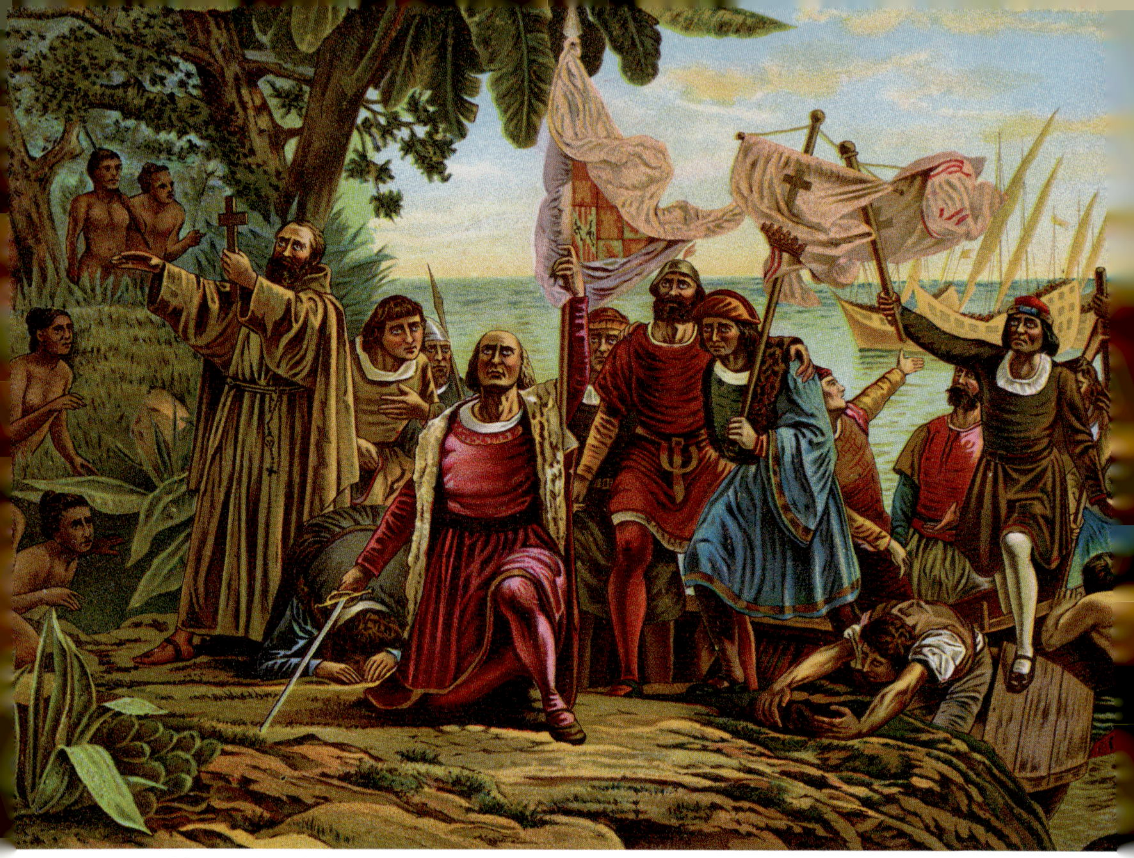

Christopher Columbus reaches land in the Americas. Europeans of the fifteenth century had different ideas about privacy than did the native peoples, just as people today hold different views of privacy than did their ancestors just a century ago.

to protect certain matters."[8] Thus, governments enact laws that protect individual privacy but also allow law enforcement personnel to intrude on personal privacy for the safety of others. For example, the Patriot Act in the United States allows the government to gather and use personal information about suspected terrorists to prevent acts of violence.

Privacy laws vary in different countries, but all in some way spell out exactly what privacy rights entail, how the government protects these rights, and what the consequences are for violating these rights. The privacy laws in many countries conform to Article 12 of the 1948 United Nations Universal Declaration of Human Rights, which states, "No one shall be subjected to arbitrary interference with his privacy, family, home or correspondence, nor to attacks upon his honour and reputation. Everyone has the right to the protection of the law against such interference or attacks."[9]

American Privacy Laws

In the United States, privacy laws derive partly from the Constitution's guarantee that people have the right to protect themselves and their property from others. Although the Constitution does not mention the word "privacy," most legal scholars have determined that the right to protect oneself and one's property also applies to personal privacy. These laws also stem from the Fourth Amendment to the Constitution, which states that the government cannot intrude on anyone's home or property without a search warrant. The Fourteenth Amendment, which guarantees each American the liberty to make personal decisions, has also been interpreted to apply to privacy rights.

Several legal experts have argued that the United States does not need special privacy laws in addition to the rights already granted by the Constitution. For instance, lawyer Judith Jarvis Thompson argued in 1975 that the constitutional rights to liberty, property, and bodily security also apply to and protect privacy rights. Other legal experts believe that since the Constitution does not include the word "privacy," the founding fathers of the United States did not intend to include privacy as a basic right. One such expert, Judge Robert Bork, writes in his book *The Tempting of America* that many Supreme Court justices have invented the notion of a constitutional right to privacy to advance their own political beliefs. Most legal experts, and most American citizens, however, believe that the right to privacy is implicitly guaranteed by the Constitution and that special privacy laws are also needed.

> "Privacy is both a positive and a negative right; it is not just a freedom from the state, but also a duty of the state to protect certain matters."[8]
>
> *—George Washington University law professor Daniel J. Solove.*

Specific privacy laws have been enacted throughout the history of the United States to keep pace with social and technological changes. For instance, in the eighteenth century post office workers often read mail addressed to others because at that time letters were difficult to seal. This made people wary of including confidential information in letters sent through the post office. Many people, including George Washington and Thomas Jefferson, wrote letters in code to keep the contents private. Based on this issue, the US Congress enacted laws to ensure the privacy of mail. To encourage compliance with these laws, Benjamin Franklin, who served as postmaster general from 1753–1776, required postal employees to take an oath that they would not open other peoples' mail.

After the invention of the telegraph in 1844, privacy issues about telegraphed messages emerged. Western Union, the company that transmitted telegrams, required its employees to keep messages confidential. State and federal laws were also enacted to prohibit people from intercepting telegrams and to prohibit the government from accessing private telegrams except in criminal investigations.

The invention of the telephone in 1876 forced privacy laws to evolve further. Wiretapping technologies that allowed people to listen in on phone conversations emerged in the 1890s. Early laws allowed wiretapping, but by 1968 these laws had all been amended to prohibit wiretapping except in cases where law enforcement personnel had a warrant signed by a court.

Expanding Privacy Laws in the 1900s

When newspapers began using newly invented handheld cameras and new printing technologies to print pictures and stories about newsworthy people in the late 1800s, this spurred attorney Samuel Warren and Supreme Court justice Louis Brandeis to write an essay titled "The Right to Privacy." The article appeared in the *Harvard Law Review* in 1890. In their essay Warren and Brandeis call privacy "the right to be let alone" and argue that the media's right to publish news does not mean they can intrude on peoples' private lives and harm peoples' reputations. An excerpt from the essay reads: "Instantaneous photographs and newspaper enterprise have invaded the sacred precincts of private and domestic life. . . . The press is overstepping in every direction the obvious bounds of propriety and of decency . . . the individual is entitled to decide whether that which is his shall be given to the public. . . . It is

> "The individual is entitled to decide whether that which is his shall be given to the public."[10]
>
> *—Nineteenth-century attorney Samuel Warren and Supreme Court justice Louis Brandeis.*

The Origins of the Internet

Many threats to health care privacy in the online world occur when electronic medical records are accessed through the Internet. The concept that led to the development of the Internet originated in 1969 with the ARPANET (Advanced Research Projects Agency Network) project. ARPANET set up a network of computers around the world that allowed information to flow securely between US military bases. It was designed by a group of computer experts who incorporated the idea of the "Galactic Network" and the concept of "packet switches" into a network of computers that could communicate.

J.C.R. Licklider of the Massachusetts Institute of Technology (MIT) introduced his Galactic Network idea in 1962. He envisioned linking computers all over the world electronically so people could share data. Lawrence Roberts of MIT advanced this idea in 1965 by connecting a computer in California to one in Massachusetts using a telephone line. He realized, however, that using telephone circuits would not allow high-speed computer networking to occur. Roberts consulted with several scientists who were working on developing packet switches as an alternative to the circuit switches in telephone lines. Packet switches group digital data into small blocks called packets. This allows data to be transmitted faster than telephone circuits allow.

Roberts was one of the scientists who incorporated the first packet switches into the ARPANET project. Later, this type of connection was used to launch the World Wide Web, or Internet. Like any technology, the Internet can be used for good or bad purposes.

like the right not to be assaulted or beaten, the right not to be imprisoned, the right not to be maliciously prosecuted, the right not to be defamed."[10]

Legal scholars consider "The Right to Privacy" to be the basis for new expansions and interpretations of privacy laws in the 1900s. Laws that regulated the power of the media to intrude on peoples' privacy were enacted after this essay was published; balancing these laws with the First Amendment's guarantee of a free press led to controversies that continue to rage in America. Many celebrities, in particular, have lamented the fact that their privacy is regularly intruded upon by aggressive reporters and photographers, despite the existence of privacy laws. Celebrities have also expressed outrage about the fact that tabloid newspapers pay people to commit these intrusions, as happened with the celebrity medical file breaches at UCLA Medical Center and elsewhere. After Lawanda Jackson was caught selling information about Farrah Fawcett to the *National Enquirer*, for example, Fawcett stated that she believed the tabloid, as well as Jackson, should be prosecuted for criminal behavior. This did not happen, however, because the First Amendment protects to a great extent the media's right to report news.

Actress Farrah Fawcett (pictured in 2005) urged criminal prosecution of a hospital employee and tabloid newspaper that obtained confidential information from her electronic health records. Hospital employees can be punished for such actions but news media have many protections.

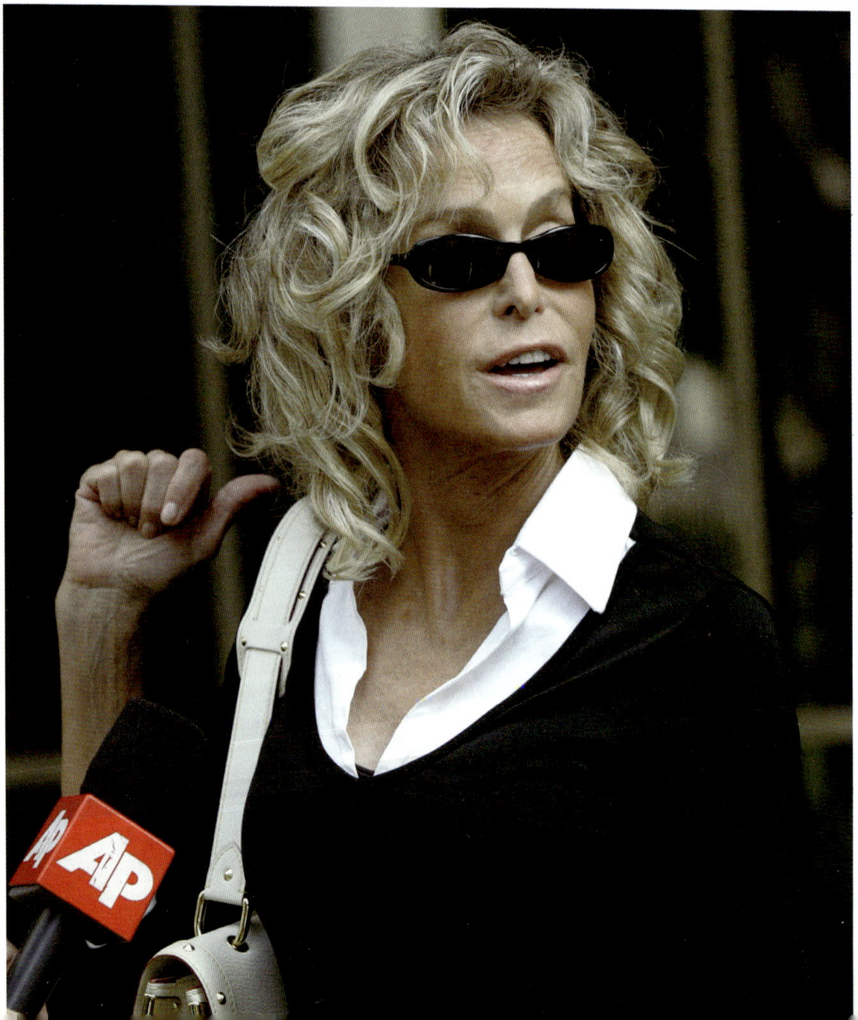

Who Values Privacy More?

Although Americans value their privacy, in general "Europe has historically been more protective of personal information than the United States, which has no general law to protect peoples' privacy while most EU [European Union] countries do," explains a *New York Times* article. Privacy experts believe this is because the United States has traditionally been more concerned about the free flow of information and the ability of private businesses to flourish than European countries are.

All twenty-seven EU nations have adopted some form of the EU Data Protection Directive of 1995, which asserts that individual privacy must be protected from governments and businesses. While the United States lacks a general privacy law, it does have specific privacy laws that govern certain types of information. Some of these specific laws are strict, while others are not. American health care privacy laws are strict, but they do allow patient data to be sold to businesses in the interests of economic growth. They also allow the government to access private data for law enforcement and national security purposes.

Many Americans believe that privacy laws of all types should be changed to give individuals more protection from business and government intrusions. A 2011 survey by Opera Software revealed that Americans overwhelmingly value their privacy and that 22 to 29 percent of the people surveyed fear online privacy invasions more than they fear terrorist attacks, bankruptcy, or criminals breaking into their homes.

New York Times, "Europe Moves Ahead on Privacy," February 3, 2013. www.nytimes.com.

Other Privacy Law Expansions

Other significant privacy law expansions occurred throughout the twentieth century. For instance, the constitutional right to privacy was expanded to include the right to make personal and family decisions. This change occurred as a result of a 1965 Supreme Court case known as *Griswold v. Connecticut*. In this case, a lower court had convicted the director of Planned Parenthood and a Yale University doctor of unlawfully sharing information about contraceptives with married couples. The Supreme Court overturned the convictions, based on the argument that the constitutional right to privacy allows people to make personal and family decisions without government interference. This meant that the government could no longer regulate whether individuals received information about contraception or chose to use contraceptive products. After this, the constitutional right to privacy was used to uphold individuals' rights to make other personal decisions. One of the most well-known personal rights guaranteed by the constitutional right to privacy since 1973 is a woman's right to have an abortion. The Supreme Court upheld this right in the historic and controversial *Roe v. Wade* case.

The Privacy Act of 1974 was another law that expanded privacy rights to keep pace with social and technological advances. The government's first computerized databases emerged in the 1960s and 1970s, and people became concerned about abuses of their electronic information. The Privacy Act of 1974 required the government to show an individual any records kept on him or her if requested by the individual. It also forbade the government from sharing any personal information without the person's consent, except for certain purposes such as law enforcement. The act also gave individuals the right to sue the government for failure to protect personal information.

"It is recognized that health information belongs to the individual who is the subject of such information. . . . Thus, use of health information always requires the consent of the individual owner."[11]

—Electronic Healthcare Information Security.

The HIPAA regulations that were first enacted in 1996 incorporated many elements of the Privacy Act of 1974. Those rules have been amended several times as evolving Internet and wireless technologies have brought about new challenges to the security of private information. However, the basic rationale behind these health care privacy laws has remained the same over time. The book *Electronic Healthcare Information Security* describes this rationale: "It is recognized that health information belongs to the individual who is the subject of such information. . . . Thus, use of health information always requires the consent of the individual owner."[11]

Unique Aspects of Health Care Privacy

As with other privacy laws, the rationale for HIPAA builds on the ideas about privacy put forth by philosophers such as Aristotle and John Locke. However, health care regulations are unique in that individuals do not have direct control over personal information they share with a doctor. Instead, people trust their doctors (and hospitals or other entities in the health field) to keep their information and medical records confidential. The importance of doctor-patient confidentiality has been acknowledged since the Greek physician Hippocrates (460–377 BCE) included it in his renowned Hippocratic

The ancient Greek physician Hippocrates (conferring with a patient) acknowledged the importance of confidentiality between doctors and patients when he wrote the Hippocratic oath. Modern medicine still adheres to this important principle.

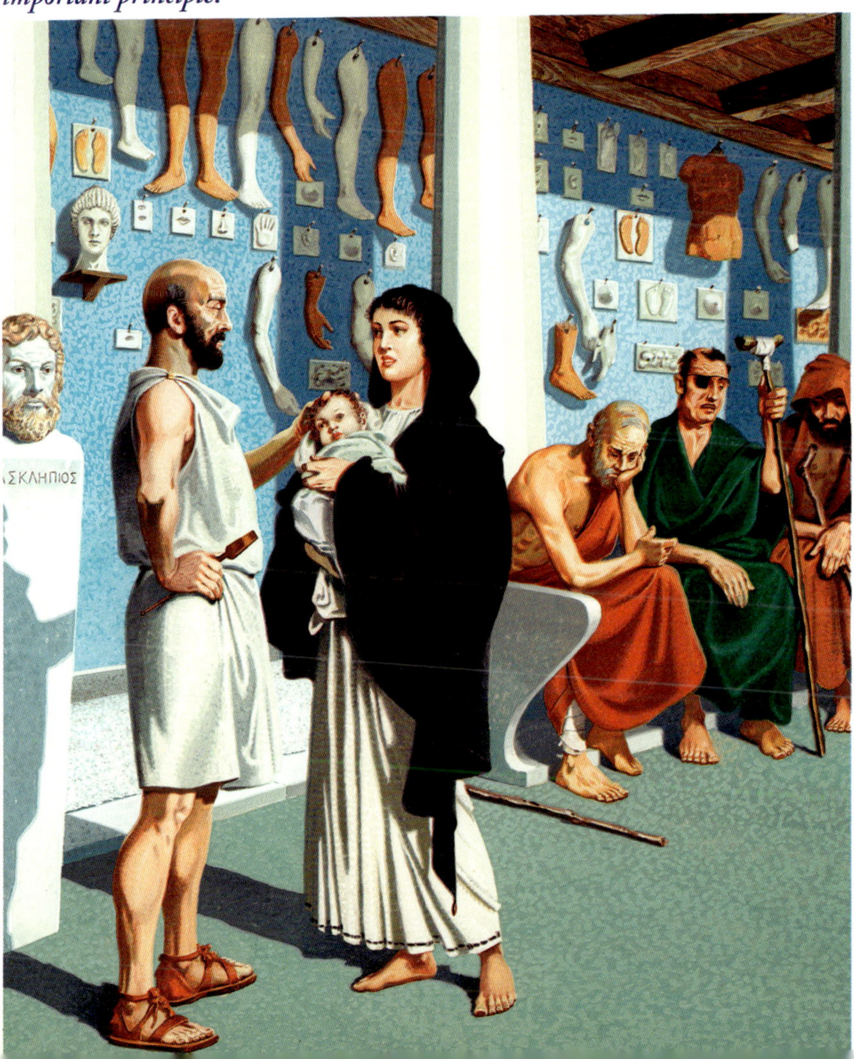

oath. Hippocrates, who is known as the father of medicine, wrote the Hippocratic oath to delineate doctors' ethical responsibilities. The section that concerns doctor-patient confidentiality states, "Whatever I see or hear in the lives of my patients, whether in connection with my professional practice or not, which ought not to be spoken of outside, I will keep secret, as considering all such things to be private."[12]

Today, doctors swear to uphold an updated version of the Hippocratic oath when they receive their medical licenses. The American Medical Association notes that "maintaining patient confidentiality is a legal duty as well as an ethical duty. . . . Any breach in confidentiality—even one that seems minor—can result in mistrust and, possibly, a lawsuit and/or disciplinary action."[13]

Although the words "privacy" and "confidentiality" are often used interchangeably, an article in the *Journal of the American Medical Informatics Association* explains that their definitions differ somewhat: "Privacy is the state of being free from intrusion. . . . Confidentiality, in contrast, is the limiting of information to only those for whom it is appropriate. . . . If someone follows you and spies on you entering an AIDS clinic, your privacy is violated; if someone who works in the clinic faxes your health care records to a newspaper reporter without your permission or knowledge, your records' confidentiality is violated."[14]

Doctor-patient confidentiality and the privacy of health information have been increasingly challenged as more and more data is stored electronically and opportunities for unauthorized viewing and abuses multiply. Personal health information encompasses elements of every type of privacy—bodily, territorial, social, informational, and communications—that humans have needed and valued throughout history. Surveys indicate that patients value the privacy and confidentiality of their health records very highly, and the health care providers who are obligated to safeguard these records constantly struggle with upholding this obligation in the online world.

Chapter 2

Who Has Access to Private Medical Information?

Because of the sensitive nature of medical information, most governments today have enacted strict health care privacy regulations designed especially to protect computerized data. Medical records used to be stored on paper in files in doctors' offices and hospitals, and patients usually paid cash for their health care. Today, however, patient data is often kept in computerized, electronically networked databases, and public or private insurance companies pay for most patient care. With these trends, the number of people who have access to patient records has increased. Doctors and hospitals collect and need access to personal health information to diagnose and treat patients. Insurance companies need access to pay for care, and other companies and organizations may need access for medical research, filling patient prescriptions, and other purposes.

The Purpose of HIPAA

The HIPAA regulations in the United States mainly control who may legitimately access personal health information. These regulations also give patients the right to consent to whom the information may be disclosed and hold the medical professionals and others who collect, view, and store the information responsible for protecting its confidentiality.

The main government agencies that formulate and enforce HIPAA rules are the Department of Health and Human Services and its Office for Civil Rights, the Office of the National Coordinator for Health Information Technology, and the Centers for Medicare and Medicaid Services. In addition, the Health Information Security and Privacy Collaboration ensures that federal and state laws on medical privacy are consistent and compatible.

HIPAA sets minimum national standards for protecting patient privacy. Prior to 1996, when the US Congress passed HIPAA, each state abided by its own health care privacy rules. Since HIPAA was enacted, US states may still adopt their own privacy standards, but these cannot be less strict than the HIPAA standards.

Over the years the HIPAA regulations have been amended to meet changing social and technological innovations. For example, some HIPAA amendments address the fact that more and more mobile smartphones and laptop computers are being lost or stolen and that hackers have developed new ways of breaching hospital and medical office computer networks. These amendments emphasize the importance of encrypting patient data so it is not recognizable to anyone who is not authorized to view it. The American Medical Association explains that encryption programs produce "a scrambled form of the original data. When a legitimate user needs to access the data, the scrambling process is reversed, and the data is restored to its original

Medical records once consisted entirely of paper files stored in doctor's offices and hospitals. Most patient information today is stored in computer databases that are accessible to insurance companies, hospitals, doctors, and other medical professionals.

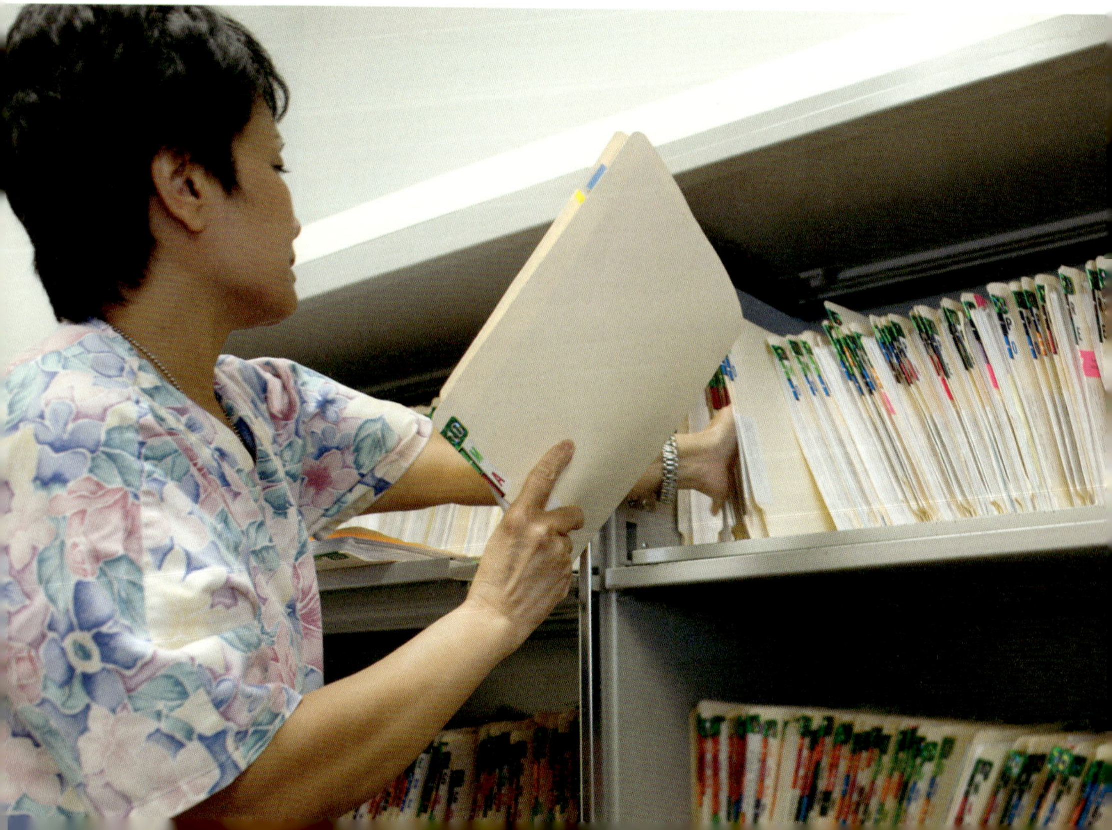

form. Only those who are in possession of the 'key' can unscramble (i.e. 'decrypt') the data."[15]

Some of the most important HIPAA changes have been legislated in the American Recovery and Reinvestment Act (ARRA) of 2009, the Health Information Technology for Economic and Clinical Health (HITECH) Act of 2009, the Affordable Care Act (ACA) of 2010, and the Omnibus Rule of 2013. All of these changes strengthen the two provisions of the HIPAA law that are most concerned with privacy. These provisions are known as the Privacy Rule and the Security Rule.

The Privacy Rule

The HIPAA Privacy Rule mandates that health care providers inform patients about their privacy rights and obtain each patient's written consent to share their medical information as needed. Patients are also asked to specify whether their information may be discussed with anyone, including family members. In addition, the Privacy Rule mandates that patients have the right to view or obtain copies of their records.

> "In practice, patients are routinely being denied the rights to simply review records."[16]
>
> *—Journalist Bernhard Warner.*

While the Privacy Rule technically gives patients the right to view their electronic health data, a 2013 survey found that 68 percent of American doctors do not believe their patients should have full access to this data. Many doctors are concerned that patients might edit the data if they can view it online. Thus, only about 20 percent of the doctors surveyed give patients access to their personal records. "In practice, patients are routinely being denied the rights to simply review records,"[16] states a *Bloomberg Businessweek* article.

Some privacy advocates are also concerned that although signing HIPAA forms is voluntary, patients actually do not have a choice. As the Privacy Rights Clearinghouse points out, "In reality, you may have no choice but to agree to the sharing of your health information if you want to obtain care and qualify for insurance."[17] Patients may also not be aware that if they are hospitalized, signing HIPAA forms means granting hundreds of people, including nurses, doctors, laboratory technicians, computer technicians, billing employees, and outside personnel in insurance companies and government permission to view their records.

Sharing Information

HIPAA also allows health care providers to share or sell patient information to companies that market products that might be beneficial to a patient. For instance, if a patient has diabetes, the health care provider can release his or her medical records, without the patient's permission, to companies that sell blood sugar monitors. However, HIPAA requires all health care providers and their employees, which the Privacy Rule calls "covered entities," and outside companies called "business associates of covered entities," to sign agreements to safeguard the confidentiality of patient information.

The requirement to safeguard patient information applies to all forms of communication—spoken, written, faxed, electronic, or other. Since many privacy breaches occur during oral conversations, many hospitals and other facilities have rules that prohibit employees from discussing patients anywhere that unauthorized people might overhear them. However, the Privacy Rule also recognizes that sometimes it is impossible to prevent confidential information from being overheard. For example, in busy hospital emergency rooms, patients are often separated by curtains that do not block sound. Some patients who are hospitalized also have roommates. In such cases, doctors are not considered to be at fault if others can overhear their private conversations with patients.

> "In reality, you may have no choice but to agree to the sharing of your health information if you want to obtain care and qualify for insurance."[17]
>
> —*The Privacy Rights Clearinghouse.*

The Privacy Rule also specifies that when health care providers do share or allow access to private health information, they must "make reasonable efforts to limit use, disclosures of, and requests for PHI [protected health information] to the minimum necessary to accomplish the intended purpose."[18] This requirement is known as the Minimum Necessary Standard. As an example, when a hospital provides treatment information to an insurance company, it usually

Britney Spears and Dr. Phil

HIPAA laws apply to licensed medical professionals and their employees, but not when they reveal information about a patient who is not under their care. The public became aware of this fact in 2008 after pop star Britney Spears was hospitalized in Los Angeles for psychiatric problems. Television psychotherapist Phil McGraw, widely known as Dr. Phil, visited Spears in the hospital at her parents' request. Afterward, he told *Entertainment Tonight* about the meeting and stated that Spears needed extensive medical and psychiatric help. Many people accused Dr. Phil of violating patient privacy laws. However, during an investigation, the state licensing board in California revealed that McGraw was not licensed in California. He was previously licensed as a clinical psychologist in Texas but never in California. This fact, plus the fact that he was not Spears's doctor and did not visit her to treat her illness, exempted him from being bound by medical privacy laws.

Spears's parents, however, stated on the *Today Show* that McGraw violated their trust when he spoke publicly about the visit. They also said that McGraw was exploiting Spears's fame to further his own television career. Lou Taylor, a Spears family spokesperson, explained, "The family basically extended an invitation of trust as a resource to support them, not to make a public statement. Any public statements he made, because he was brought in under this cloak of trust, are just inappropriate."

Quoted in Mike Celizic, "Spears' Parents Say Dr. Phil Violated Their Trust," *Today Entertainment*, January 9, 2008. www.today.com.

lists diagnostic and treatment codes with no details included unless the insurer requests further information. In other situations, such as when a doctor is required to release a patient's records in a legal matter, the doctor must use his or her discretion and release only those details that are relevant to the court case.

However, doctors who share patient information among themselves or with nurses are exempt from the Minimum Necessary Standard. This is because all doctors and nurses who help with a patient's care need full access to the medical records to do their jobs. This has created some controversy because the exemption also applies to medical and nursing students in teaching hospitals. These students are given full access to patient records to help the students learn. Students are required to understand and adhere to HIPAA privacy rules, but several surveys have found that many do not fully comprehend what privacy means. One survey found, for instance, that 60 percent of medical school deans reported that their students inappropriately posted patient-related details on Facebook, Twitter, and other social media sites. Thirteen percent of medical students actually identified patients in their postings and were found guilty of HIPAA violations. The students erroneously believed that once they left the hospital, they could post whatever they wanted on their personal sites. Some patients have requested that students not be given access to their records because of such occurrences. However, teaching hospitals do not honor these requests.

The Security Rule

Even though privacy breaches like this do happen, in most situations allowing the free flow of information among doctors and nurses is beneficial for patients because it enhances the quality of care. This is why the Privacy Rule allows personal information to be accessed by a variety of people, sometimes many more than a patient would prefer. The HIPAA Security Rule, which further regulates how patient information is to be protected, works hand in hand with the Privacy Rule to enhance patient privacy while allowing effective health care to proceed. According to the National Institute of Standards and Technology website, "The Security Rule sets federal standards to protect the confidentiality, integrity and availability of electronic protected health information by requiring HIPAA covered entities and their business associates to implement and maintain administrative, physical and technical safeguards."[19] This means that these organizations and businesses must guard their computers and put appropriate computer software and employee training programs in place. They must also sign contracts agreeing to follow HIPAA rules.

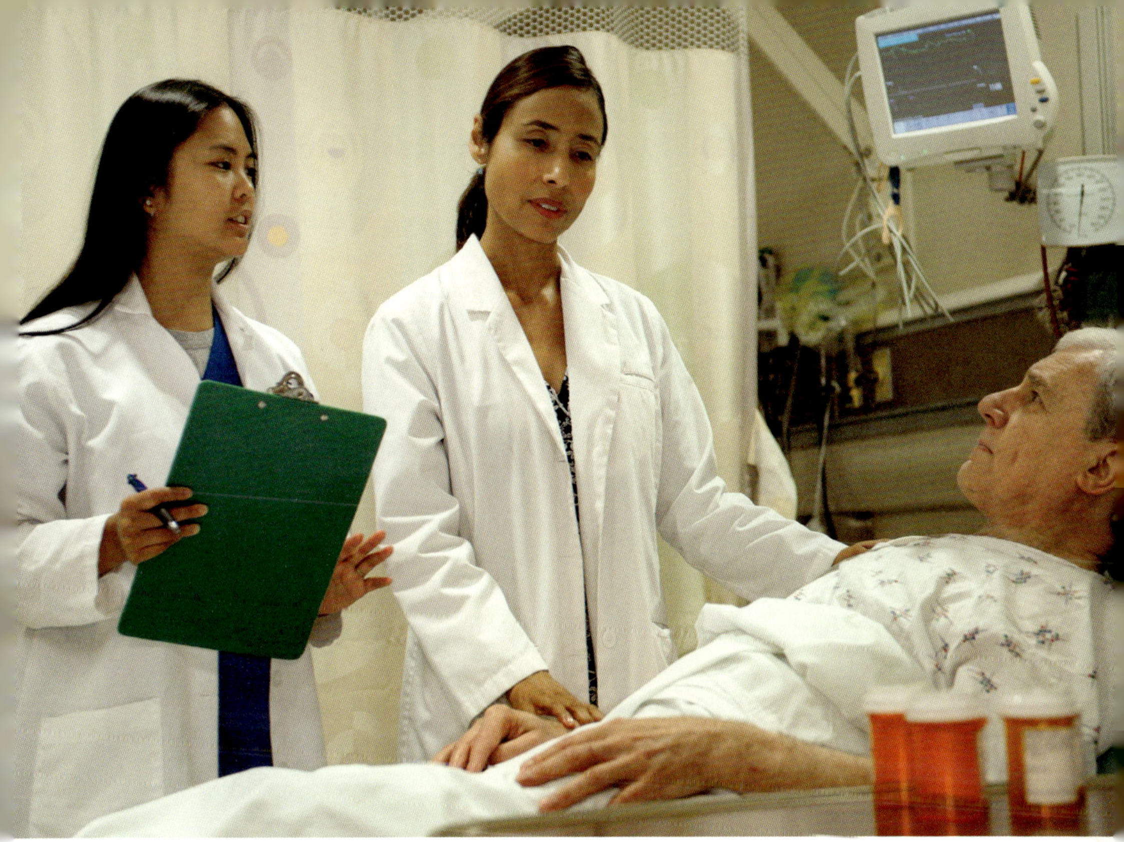

Federal law requires caregivers to safeguard confidential patient information, but it also recognizes that doctor-patient conversations might be overheard in settings such as emergency rooms where patients are separated by curtains rather than doors.

When health care providers and other covered entities share or sell patient information to business associates that have signed HIPAA contracts, all identifying information about patients can be included. For example, medical insurance companies send complete patient information to the Medical Information Bureau and pharmacies send it to IntelliScript and MedPoint. These are business associates that keep databases about patients' medical histories and use of prescription medications. If someone applies for a medical or life insurance policy, IntelliScript and MedPoint then provide information on the individual's prescription drug use and health status to underwriters who decide whether to approve these applications.

In some instances the Security Rule allows covered entities to share or sell patient information to companies that are not considered to be business associates. Most of the time, under HIPAA's Safe Harbor Rule, these records will not contain patient names or other identifying

Genetic Privacy Scandal in Minnesota

HIPAA and other federal laws specifically protect the privacy of genetic information, and many states have their own genetic privacy laws as well. In Minnesota genetic privacy is protected by the Minnesota Genetic Privacy Act. An April 2013 article in the *St. Paul Pioneer Press* revealed that officials in the Minnesota Department of Public Health have been violating this law for several decades by illegally storing, using, and sharing newborns' genetic data without the knowledge or permission of the children's parents.

After the Minnesota Supreme Court ruled that the state's Department of Health was guilty of these violations, the department began a campaign to influence the state legislature to pass a bill that would legalize storing, using, and sharing genetic data without permission. The proposed bill would also extend back to the time when these practices started so those responsible could not be punished. According to the newspaper article, "They now want the Legislature to retroactively legalize what they did—and let them keep doing it in the future."

Whether or not the bill will pass remains to be seen.

St. Paul Pioneer Press, "'Biobank' Bill Threatens Genetic Privacy," April 17, 2013. www.cchfreedom.org.

information. Health information experts call this "de-identifying" the records. Public health agencies, however, are exempt from the Safe Harbor Rule. They are allowed to sell identifiable hospital records to data-mining companies or others to earn money. Data-mining companies collect and store information about individuals and resell the information to businesses such as drug companies, which then advertise their products to these individuals.

When patient information is not sold by public health agencies, identification details must be deleted if the buyer is not a HIPAA-covered business associate. However, sometimes these companies, particularly those that perform health research, need to know who each patient is. In such cases the researchers generally ask patients to grant permission for their identities to be included in the research databases. When this is impossible, as in instances where a research participant is deceased, HIPAA rules allow a research institution's privacy board to authorize the use of identifying data if the benefits to society outweigh the risks to a patient's privacy. A National Institutes of Health publication explains that these rules seek to balance individual privacy rights with the common good: "The primary justification for protecting personal privacy is to protect the interests of individuals. In contrast, the primary justification for collecting personally identifiable health information for health research is to benefit society."[20]

Where Else Is Information Shared?

Doctors and hospitals may also be compelled to share identifiable patient information in other instances where the common good is at stake. For example, doctors are required to report all gunshot injuries and instances of suspected physical abuse to police so the victim and others can be protected and the perpetrator punished. Doctors must also disclose patient information to law enforcement personnel to prevent acts of violence. If a psychiatrist treats a patient who threatens to kill others, for example, the doctor is obligated to notify police and the individuals who have been threatened.

> "The primary justification for protecting personal privacy is to protect the interests of individuals. In contrast, the primary justification for collecting personally identifiable health information for health research is to benefit society."[20]
>
> —*National Institutes of Health.*

Physicians are also required to disclose patients' names and medical records to public health departments when a patient has a contagious disease. In such cases, public health departments must warn others who are at risk of becoming infected. This issue often arises when a patient is diagnosed with a sexually transmitted disease such as AIDS (Acquired Immune Deficiency Syndrome). Many states have laws that give people who have AIDS or who test positive for HIV (human immunodeficiency virus), the virus that causes AIDS, special privacy protections. This is because of past discrimination against HIV-positive people in housing, employment, and insurance eligibility. However, public health departments are also required to ask patients with AIDS or HIV to identify all their sexual partners. The health department then informs these partners that they should be tested for the disease. In such cases, the law views the section of the Hippocratic oath that reads, "I will prevent disease whenever I can, for prevention is preferable to cure"[21] as being more important than doctor-patient confidentiality because public health is at risk.

Discrimination has also affected people who receive genetic tests that indicate they may develop certain types of cancer and other genetically linked diseases. Ever since scientists sequenced the human genome (the complete set of human DNA) in 2004, many people have undergone genetic tests to find out whether they are likely to develop certain illnesses or to pass abnormal genes to their offspring. In some cases, employers who saw the test results would not hire an individual or even fired an employee. Insurance companies also would not insure people with some genetic abnormalities. For this reason, Congress passed the Genetic Information Nondiscrimination Act (GINA) in 2008. GINA prohibits discrimination based on genetic information and prohibits employers and insurers from asking about or gaining access to this information. HIPAA rules also protect the privacy of genetic information.

Another special class of protected health information that is covered by both HIPAA and other laws is injuries or illnesses resulting from an individual's job. Such information must be kept separate, in an occupational medical record, from the person's other health records. According to Occupational Safety and Health Administration (OSHA) rules, doctors who treat occupational medical problems are obligated to send patients' occupational records to the employer, OSHA, and the patient's regular doctor. These records must adhere strictly to HIPAA's Minimum Necessary Standard. The American Health Information Management Association explains that "the healthcare provider needs to 'make reasonable efforts' to ensure that only the minimum amount of information is disclosed to achieve the intended purpose. This is important when the healthcare provider is conducting an evaluation for a specified limited purpose and the patient discloses other unrelated PHI."[22] In other words, if

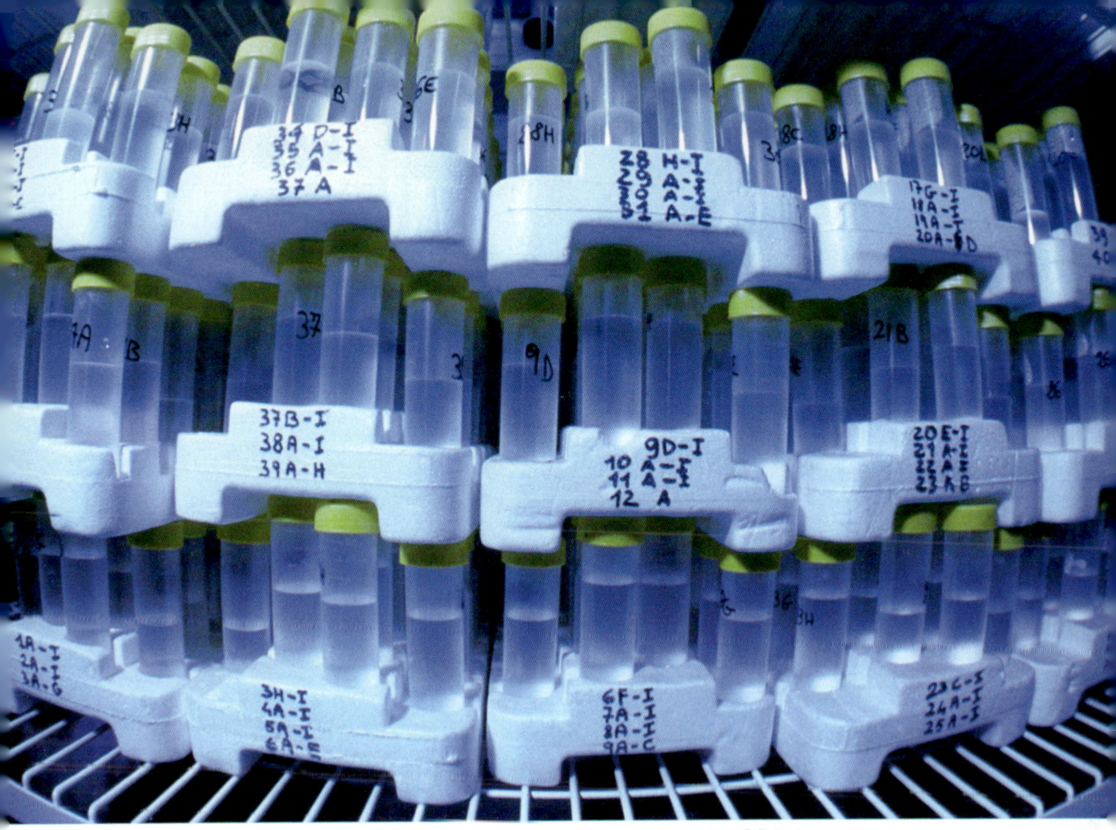

Test tubes in a gene bank laboratory contain segments of DNA that make up the entire human genome. Genetic tests made possible by the sequencing of the human genome are protected under federal privacy rules.

a patient breaks a leg while working for a construction company, the doctor who treats the leg may not include information in the occupational medical record about the patient's additional complaint of being depressed.

Flexibility in HIPAA Rules

Revealing the minimum amount of information in work-related and other situations is one example of how HIPAA sometimes gives health care providers discretion to use their own judgment. Another example relates to sharing patient information with family members, friends, or others directly involved in caring for a patient at home or in paying for their care. Many times, a patient does not give specific permission for a provider to share information with these individuals. According to the Department of Health and Human Services, "The covered entity may share relevant information with the family and these other persons if it can reasonably infer, based on professional judgment, that the patient does not object."[23]

For example, a doctor may reasonably infer that a patient would not object if a friend who will be staying with the patient after a hospitalization is informed about the patient's medication dosages. By the same token, a pharmacist may deem it to be permissible to discuss side effects of a prescribed medication with a family member who is purchasing the medication for a patient.

HIPAA rules also give doctors discretion in decisions not to share patient information with a family member or friend. This might happen in a situation where the doctor believes the family member or friend has been abusive to the patient. Such a decision can apply to adults or children. Thus, if a doctor suspects that a parent is abusing a child, that doctor may choose to withhold information from the parent and may petition a court to make medical decisions that the parent would normally make for the child.

The HIPAA rules are complex and allow these types of exceptions because medical care and privacy are complex. While privacy laws usually override other considerations, sometimes the safety of patients or others is viewed as being more important than privacy.

Chapter 3

The Push for Electronic Medical Records

Although many health care providers already use computerized medical records, nearly half of all doctors in the United States still used paper charts and other paper records in 2012. The medical field has been slower than most other industries to adopt electronic record keeping for several reasons. One reason is that the unique nature of doctor-patient confidentiality compels doctors to take special measures to guard patient privacy. It is much easier to protect paper records than electronic ones, since paper records can be locked up. While breaches in paper records do occur, breaches in electronic records happen more often because these records can be accessed online or through networked computers in medical practices and hospitals.

Questions of Efficiency and Quality

Another reason many health care providers have resisted converting to electronic medical records (EMRs) is that they believe health care should not be run like a typical business. The business world values efficiency, but many doctors believe that good patient care is more important than efficiency. Many health information specialists, along with the US government, are promoting EMRs because they view this as a way to increase efficiency as well as enhance quality of care. For example, information technology expert Stephan Kudyba writes in *Healthcare Informatics*, "With the aid of accurate and timely information, and the ability to communicate and apply that information, physicians, nurses, technicians, and administrators can improve the process of caring for those in need in a more efficient, less costly manner."[24]

Many doctors who have switched to EMRs and their patients complain that even if EMRs are more efficient, they do not improve and may even diminish the quality of care. A RAND Corporation survey released in October 2013, for example, revealed that 40 percent of physicians who have switched to EMRs believe EMRs have not improved patient care. Thirty-six percent believe that using EMRs interferes with doctor-patient communication during office visits. As one doctor writes: "It's a horrible and costly bureaucracy that is being imposed on doctors. I spend less time with patients, and more time filling out multiple boxes on forms that don't fit the way I work."[25]

The RAND survey also indicated that only 18 percent of the physicians surveyed prefer paper records. Doctors such as Michael Gilbert of Orange, California, believe that paper records cannot compete with EMRs. He states: "The ability to share trends and engage the patient in their care is just light years above what we could do with paper."[26] Many patients participating in a 2013 study published in the *Journal of Medical Internet Research* state that they believe EMRs enhance health care by making it easy to view laboratory results online, streamlining prescription filling, and making medical records easily accessible when they go on vacation and must see a doctor outside their home area.

Promoting Electronic Medical Records

Among doctors who have not adopted EMRs, the most common reason is the cost, which can reach around $200,000 for computer hardware, software, and employee training. However, the US government has been promoting the use of EMRs since 2009 and is offering monetary incentives to achieve this goal. The 2009 HITECH Act provides nearly $21 billion for the government to distribute to health care providers who adopt electronic record keeping and tie in to electronic health information-sharing exchanges by 2016. Each doctor or medical practice that complies can receive up to $50,000 toward the cost of implementing any of the thousands of available EMR computer programs.

Doctors and hospitals that do not comply with the government's program will be penalized starting in 2017, when the government

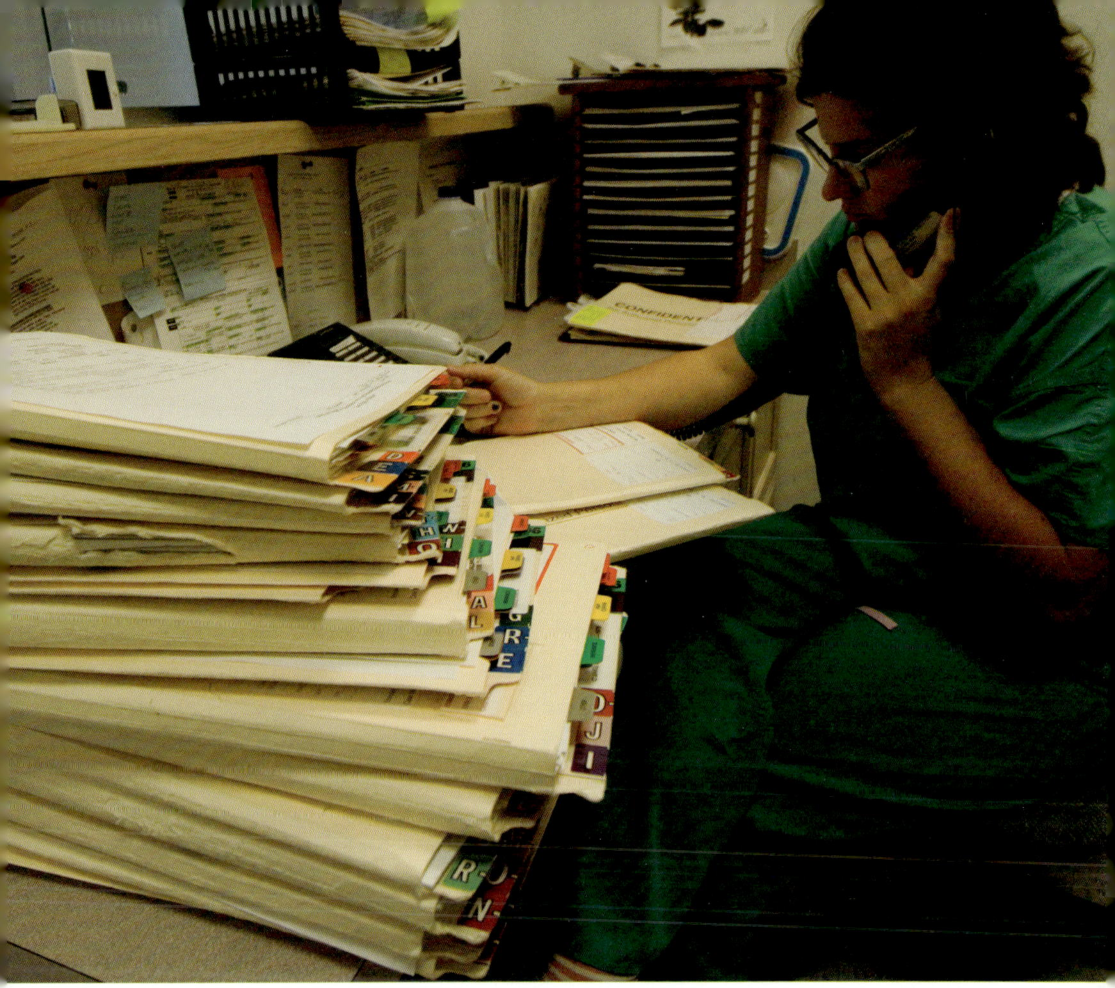

A stack of paper files awaits a nurse's attention. Nearly half of all doctors in the United States still used paper charts and records in 2012.

plans to reduce Medicare and Medicaid payments to these providers. Medicare is the federal program that pays for medical care for people over age sixty-five and for those with certain disabilities. Medicaid is the program that pays for medical care for the poor. Because of the incentives and penalties, many doctors and hospitals have switched to EMRs over the past few years, and others plan to do so before the deadline.

Federal officials are promoting EMRs because they believe this will improve patient safety, cut health care costs, and improve overall efficiency. In a National Public Radio interview, Farzad Mostashari, former national coordinator for health information technology, stresses the safety aspects, stating, "Electronic prescribing, ordering medications through a computer that can tell you there's a drug-drug

Interconnected Electronic Records

Many people are concerned about the US government's push for electronic medical records and for a huge Data Hub of interconnected data about individuals that can be accessed by numerous government departments. Although the potential privacy abuses are not funny, the following excerpt from humorist Dave Barry's book *Dave Barry in Cyberspace* offers a somewhat exaggerated look at what can result from centralized, interconnected databases. Barry writes about a hypothetical situation in which a man experiences a heart attack and is rushed to the hospital. Doctors administer tests, and the results are transmitted "to a giant medical database computer a thousand miles away. Almost instantaneously an electronic message comes back, informing the doctors that the patient—whom the computer has mistaken for another man with a similar name, who actually died thirty-eight months earlier—has fallen behind in his car payments and should be denied credit at the hospital. The computer then—*without even having to be asked*—disconnects the patient's electrical and phone services and cancels every one of his credit cards. All of this is accomplished in less time than it takes you to burp."

Dave Barry, *Dave Barry in Cyberspace*. New York: Ballantine, 1997, pp. 8–9.

interaction is safer than hand-scrawling it on paper. . . . The best thing we can do for patient safety is to get off paper."[27]

Patient Safety

Several reports indicate that using EMRs significantly enhances patient safety. Medical errors that result in patient harm or death have been an ongoing problem in hospitals and other health care facilities for many years. According to the National Coordinating Council for Medication Error Reporting and Prevention, about 98,000 people in the United States die each year due to medication errors alone. Switching to EMRs has been shown to reduce the incidence of these errors, in part by coordinating care among providers and allowing them immediate access to newly updated records. Other times, errors are reduced when EMRs flag possible adverse interactions among medications or changes in patients' vital signs or laboratory test results. Another way in which EMRs reduce errors is that many errors result from nurses, pharmacists, and other doctors not being able to read doctors' handwriting in paper charts and prescriptions. Many hospitals that switch to EMRs report large reductions in overall errors. North Shore University Health System in Illinois, for instance, reported an 80 percent reduction in 2012. A community hospital in Vermont reported a 60 percent decrease in medication errors after they switched to EMRs.

While EMRs can enhance overall patient safety, a 2012 report by the Institute of Medicine indicates that sometimes human errors in entering diagnostic and treatment codes into computers lead to deadly mistakes. Patients have been given the wrong medications and even the wrong surgical procedures because of such errors. In several cases where parts of EMRs were accidently deleted, patients did not receive medications or procedures they were supposed to receive. The report concludes that many adverse medical consequences of EMRs occur when health care professionals are not properly trained or do not use information technology correctly: "The way in which health IT is designed, implemented, and used can determine whether it is an effective tool for improving patient safety or a hindrance that threatens patient safety and causes patient harm."[28] As an example, when a pediatric intensive care unit at a Pittsburgh hospital started using a new electronic health record system, their patient mortality (death) rate increased. On the other hand, the mortality rate decreased at a Seattle pediatric hospital that purchased the same system, probably as a result of better employee training on the system's use.

> "The best thing we can do for patient safety is to get off paper."[27]
>
> —*Former National Coordinator for Health Information Technology Farzad Mostashari.*

The Data Hub and Patient Privacy

In addition to patient safety concerns, many health care professionals and privacy advocates are concerned that the US government's promotion of EMRs will erode patient privacy, especially since this promotion coincides with the full rollout of the Affordable Care Act (ACA). The main purpose of the ACA (also known as Obamacare) is to help people who lack medical insurance obtain it through affordable insurance exchanges. The law mandates that every American must have medical insurance or face penalties. Those who earn less than a certain amount are eligible for government subsidies or other assistance.

A pharmacist seeks clarification on a handwritten prescription from a doctor. Electronic medical records have reduced the number of errors in prescriptions and hospital care.

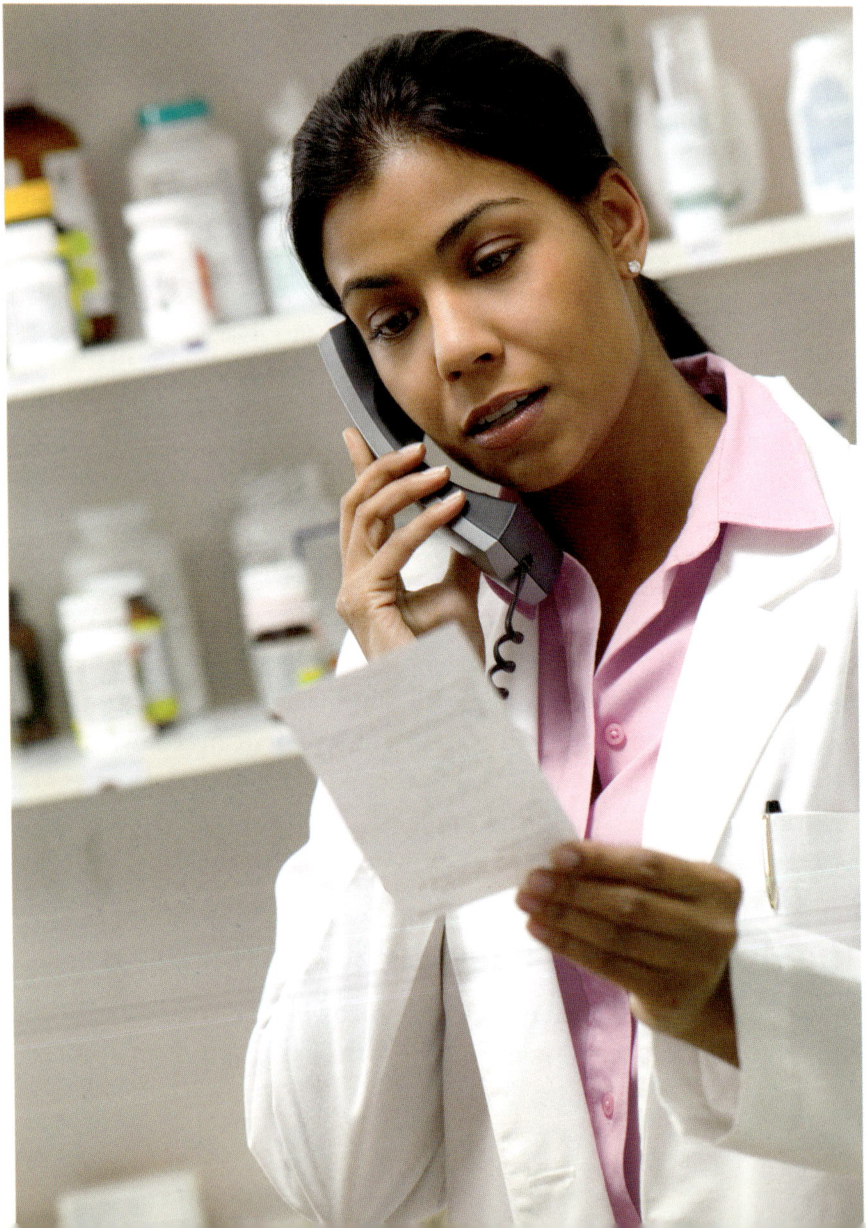

The aspect of Obamacare that experts view as most troubling from a privacy standpoint is the new Data Hub that electronically links hospitals, doctors' offices, and health care systems with government departments. The Department of Health and Human Services (HHS) states that the Data Hub will not store information and exists only to route information to appropriate government departments. However, the security of the Data Hub and the federal Healthcare.gov website, where individuals can sign up for the new insurance exchanges, has been widely questioned.

In addition, the fact that the Internal Revenue Service (IRS) is responsible for determining who is eligible for subsidies and for enforcing the mandate to purchase insurance is also of concern. To achieve this mission, the IRS has access through the Data Hub to Americans' financial information, family size information, and insurance coverage data. They may also share this information with other federal agencies such as Homeland Security and the Social Security Administration so these agencies can check citizenship status. Many people are alarmed about the IRS playing a role in Obamacare because the agency has abused its authority in the past. In one ongoing case, the IRS and fifteen of its agents are being sued for violating HIPAA privacy laws and the Fourth Amendment to the Constitution in March 2011. The fifteen agents seized 60 million personal EMRs from a California health care company without a warrant.

Security Concerns

Security concerns about the Data Hub and Healthcare.gov website were heightened during the last week of September 2013, just before Americans could start signing up for insurance through the new exchanges. An internal memo at the Centers for Medicare and Medicaid Services revealed that a security assessment on the website and Data Hub had not been completed because of pressures to launch the program on schedule on October 1. The memo indicated there was a high security risk for personal information placed in the system. For these reasons, some privacy experts and politicians urged a halt to implementing the ACA, but the program began as planned in October 2013.

The problem of inadequate security measures surfaced with reports of privacy breaches in November 2013. On November 5, 2013, South Carolina attorney Tom Dougall reported that the HealthCare.gov website breached his privacy by sharing his personal information with another website user. Justin Hadley of North Carolina contacted Dougall to let him know that he found the information about Dougall in a letter posted to Hadley's Healthcare.gov account. In another case, on November 9, 2013, HHS informed Lisa Martinson of Missouri that three unauthorized Healthcare.gov users were given access to Martinson's Social Security number, home address, and other personal information. After the Dougall incident, Medicare chief Marilyn Tavenner told a Senate committee that a software fix was made immediately. Tavenner and HHS secretary Kathleen Sebelius also pointed out that any large-scale digital undertaking involves glitches and that all the security and other problems with the ACA website would soon be fixed.

Government Intrusions

Even when the security protections for the Data Hub and Healthcare.gov website become fully operational, many privacy advocates are concerned that the Data Hub will still give the government unlimited authority to snoop in Americans' private lives. The fact that the federal Data Hub is linked to state government databases, allowing the federal and state governments to share information about peoples' income, family size, citizenship, health status, and other private data, has also led privacy advocates to complain. One article on the America's Watchtower website states, "The Data Hub will provide web-based one-stop shopping for prying into people's personal affairs."[29] America's Watchtower is a conservative advocacy group that believes the US government interferes too often in peoples' lives.

> "The Data Hub will provide web-based, one-stop shopping for prying into peoples' personal affairs."[29]
>
> *—The conservative advocacy group America's Watchtower website.*

In response to such concerns, several government agencies and numerous health care and legal experts have pointed out that the government already has access to Americans' personal information. A July 2013 CNN article, for example, states that HHS already "stores and shares personal information electronically, and has extensive safeguards in place. . . . The IRS [already] provides access to tax-return information over the Internet to nearly 300 federal and

Personal Health Record Storage

In addition to medical provider-based electronic health records, individuals can also store their medical records with online personal health records services such as Microsoft's Health Vault or Dossia. Google also ran a service called Google Health from 2008 to 2011 but discontinued it because few people used it.

Many individuals like personal health record services because they allow all their health records from different doctors to be merged into one online location. People can then share the records with doctors or others of their choosing. Many people, however, are wary of using personal health record services because they are afraid of security breaches, despite the fact that the services advertise excellent security features.

Security experts have also expressed concerns. Don Jackson, an expert in threat intelligence at Secure Works, states in an article in *SC Magazine*, "It's not a question of how good the security is. When you put all this information in one central location like this, a single compromise will affect a lot of data. . . . It's a soft target that turns out to be a treasure trove of information."

Quoted in Sue Marquette Poremba, "Privacy Issues Loom over Google Health," *SC Magazine*, May 20, 2008. www.scmagazine.com.

state agencies."[30] The article emphasizes that federal programs such as Medicare and Medicaid have had access to peoples' financial and medical care information for many years and have done a good job of protecting peoples' privacy. Additionally, the IRS and other government agencies must abide by the Privacy Act of 1974. Under this law, they must protect the security of personal information whether they are administering the tax laws or routing information through the ACA Data Hub. Thus, government officials believe Americans have no need to be alarmed about the new agency links in the Data Hub.

Numerous news and opinion articles have stated that many of the individuals who express grave concerns about the Data Hub and the

ACA in general are doing so because they wish to see the program halted. Many of these individuals have also been accused of spreading rumors about Obamacare to advance their own agendas. An October 2013 article in *Time* magazine states that many distortions of facts have resulted in public confusion about many aspects of Obamacare. The article states, "There's been so much hyperbolic nonsense written about the Affordable Care Act that it's hard to discern what's really happening."[31] The article goes on to say that even though peoples' concerns about privacy and security are valid, the hype over other issues has led many people to disregard the possible benefits of ACA once the security problems are resolved.

Additional Threats to Privacy

Along with privacy concerns about ACA and the government's push for electronic health records, several related trends have emerged that also impact patient privacy. One problem hospitals and other health providers encounter with large amounts of electronic data is that storing the data and constantly updating computer security takes up a great deal of hard drive space and employees' time. Thus, many providers store their data with outside companies called cloud service providers. According to the Center for Democracy & Technology, "Cloud computing can offer increased computing speed, capacity, flexibility, and security at significantly lower cost."[32]

> "There's been so much hyperbolic nonsense written about the Affordable Care Act that it's hard to discern what's really happening."[31]
>
> —*Time magazine journalist Joe Klein.*

HIPAA allows health care providers to store their EMRs with cloud servers and considers these companies to be business associates of the providers. Cloud companies must therefore agree to protect patient privacy. However, HHS recommends that providers not use cloud services such as Google Cloud Datastore or Dropbox that can be accessed by the public over the Internet. Instead, they recommend using private cloud storage, even though it is more expensive, because patient records are not accessible online. HHS has in fact taken legal action against health care providers that use public access cloud companies.

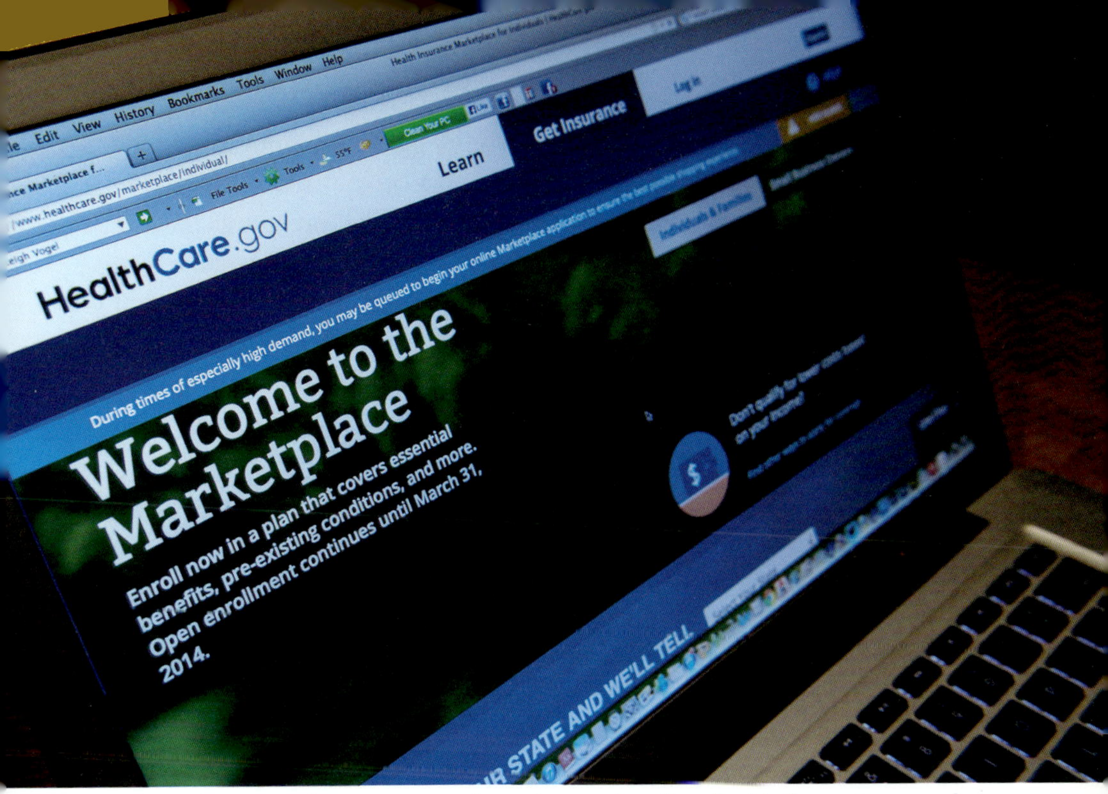

Many Americans have concerns about the security of medical information stored on the Healthcare.gov website's Data Hub. Healthcare.gov is the online federal marketplace for obtaining health insurance.

For example, in 2012 HHS fined Phoenix Cardiac Surgery $100,000 for violating HIPAA privacy and security rules when it posted information about patients' appointments on an online cloud service.

Another potential threat to patient privacy has resulted from health care providers hiring workers in foreign countries to work with their EMRs because the costs are less. This practice is known as outsourcing. US health privacy laws cannot be enforced outside the country, so providers have no way of protecting patient privacy if they employ anyone who does not live in the United States.

The University of California–San Francisco (UCSF) Medical Center found out about the dangers of outsourcing when it hired a Sausalito, California, company called Transcription Stat to transcribe their medical records. Medical records transcriptionists listen to audio recordings of doctors' notes on patient visits and enter the information into electronic databases. UCSF Medical Center was unaware that Transcription Stat was outsourcing part of their work to a transcriber in Pakistan named Lubna Baloch—until Baloch sent

UCSF an e-mail stating that she would post confidential patient medical records online unless she was paid a certain amount of money. This is known as blackmail or extortion. UCSF personnel gave in to Baloch's demands to prevent a privacy disaster. The university also terminated its contract with Transcription Stat, which went out of business. According to the American Transcription Association, a professional organization for medical transcriptionists, many health care providers continue to outsource their work despite the risk.

Hurdles for Electronic Health Records

Because of the many privacy, cost, and quality of care concerns, experts say the US government's push for the universal use of EMRs will face resistance from health care providers and patients until these problems are overcome. Studies have shown that many patients are so concerned about health care privacy risks, particularly risks related to EMRs, that they avoid seeking medical care. A 2010 HHS report revealed, for example, that nearly six hundred thousand Americans failed to seek early cancer treatment, more than 2 million did not seek mental health treatment, and many millions of young people did not seek treatment for sexually transmitted diseases because of privacy concerns.

Even though many people avoid seeking medical care for privacy reasons, however, recent surveys find that more than 80 percent of patients like many things about EMRs and believe they can improve health care. An equal number of patients are concerned about the privacy and security of their EMRs, but not to the extent that they favor paper records. The researchers who conducted one study concluded that "participants appeared willing to make tradeoffs, accepting the potential risk of breaches to their personal privacy for the convenience and accessibility of electronic records."[33]

Chapter 4

Health Care Privacy Breaches and Their Effects

Privacy concerns about electronic medical records stem from the many breaches that have occurred. A breach is defined as unauthorized use of, disclosure of, or access to private information. Health care privacy can be breached in many ways, with a variety of consequences for affected people.

Although most health care privacy breaches occur with electronic records, this is not always the case. Many nonelectronic breaches involve carelessness, as in instances where pharmacists accidently leave patient prescriptions in areas where other customers can see them or doctors discuss patients while in elevators or waiting rooms where they can be overheard. In one major breach in 2011, Massachusetts General Hospital paid the US government $1 million in fines after a hospital employee who was carrying paper medical records accidently left the records on a subway. The records were never found.

Many, many more privacy breaches, however, involve electronic data. OCR reports that nearly 23 million people's EMRs were breached between 2009 and 2012 in the United States. According to Avi Rubin, this immense number results from widespread inattention to security in the health care field. "If our financial industry regarded security the way the health-care sector does, I would stuff my cash in a mattress under my bed,"[34] Rubin states.

Theft and Carelessness

The leading cause of these privacy breaches is the theft of electronic devices, and the second leading cause is unauthorized access to and use of patient data. In many cases involving theft, computer hard drives, data sticks that store files outside a computer, or laptops have been stolen. In one instance, the theft of a hard drive from a computer in Alaska's Department of Health led to a fine of $1.7 million because OCR determined that the health department did not protect patient files well enough. Many cases in which laptop computers were stolen also led to significant penalties. In 2006, for instance, a laptop containing health files on military veterans was stolen from a data analyst's home. Although the FBI found the stolen computer and announced that no one had accessed the data, the affected veterans were awarded $20 million because of the emotional stress the incident caused.

> "If our financial industry regarded security the way the health-care sector does, I would stuff my cash in a mattress under my bed."[34]
>
> —*Computer security expert Avi Rubin.*

In a similar case in 2011, backup data tapes containing EMRs of 4.6 million military members and their families were stolen from a data company employee's car. The tapes were never found, and there is no evidence that they were ever viewed. Despite the fact that none of the people whose records were on the tapes were actually harmed, several filed a lawsuit because their privacy rights were technically violated.

Sometimes punishable breaches result from accidents or carelessness rather than theft. In 2003 in Kentucky, for instance, an outdated state health department computer was sold for twenty-five dollars to another state government office. The new owners discovered thousands of medical files on patients with sexually transmitted diseases and realized the health department had failed to clean the hard drive before selling the computer. Similar incidents have happened in other places and have led to strict regulations about the need to clean or remove hard drives before selling or disposing of computers.

Breaches Involving Online Postings

Other instances of careless privacy breaches involve online postings rather than physical equipment. In one major breach in 2010–2011, information about twenty thousand emergency room patients at Stanford University Hospital was posted on a spreadsheet on the

Student of Fortune website for nearly a year. This website provides paid help with schoolwork for students. The spreadsheet containing patient names, billing information, and medical details was placed on the site by a billing company job applicant who sought help with converting the spreadsheet to a graph. According to a *New York Times* article, "Although medical security breaches are not uncommon, the Stanford breach was notable for the length of time that the data remained publicly available without detection."[35] After a patient discovered the posting, the hospital immediately had it removed and offered free identity protection to affected people. They also stopped working with the billing company that was responsible for the breach. Even though Stanford was not directly responsible, the affected patients sued both Stanford and the billing company for $20 million because under HIPAA, a health care provider is responsible for ensuring that its business associates enforce security measures.

Another serious online breach occurred when the University of Chicago Medical Center published an online manual for residents

Some hospital employees have posted photos and comments about patients on social media sites. Employees can be fired for such actions, as most hospitals have rules against breaching patient privacy in this way.

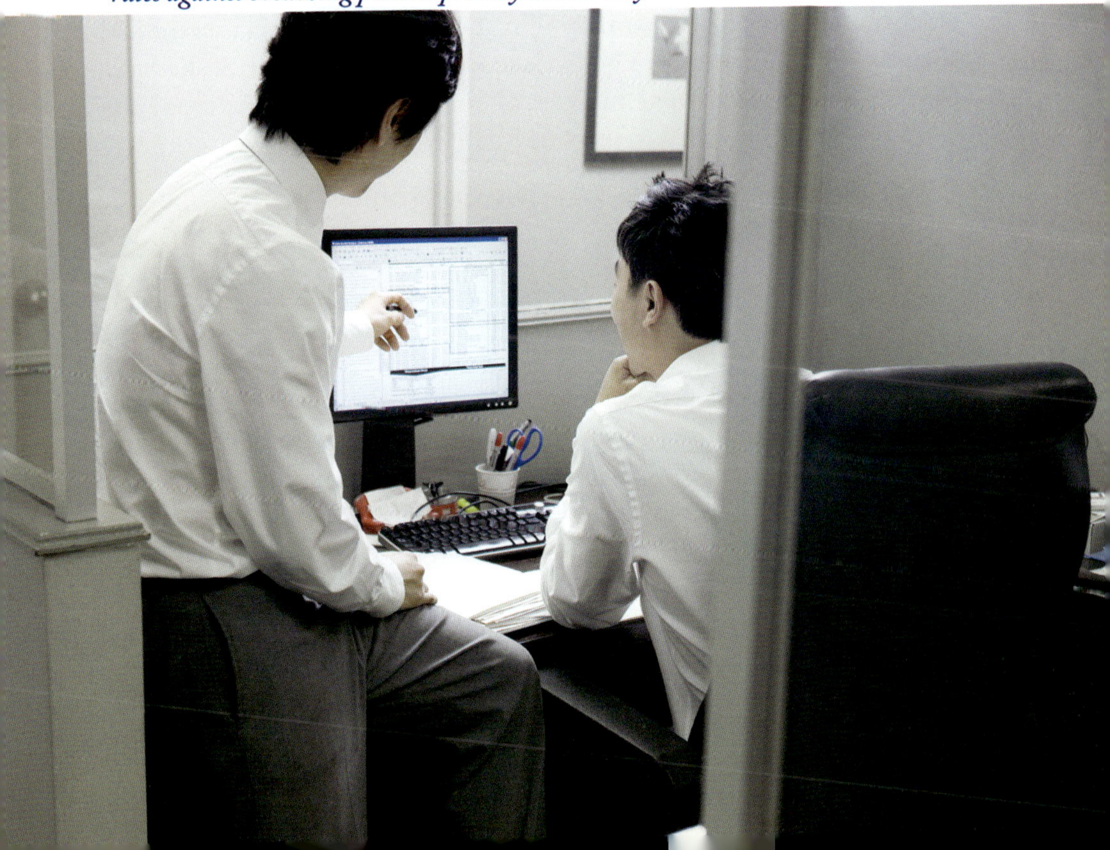

A Nonelectronic Privacy Breach

While most health information privacy breaches occur with electronic data, some still happen in other ways. One of the best known of such breaches occurred in December 2012 in England after Catherine, wife of Prince William, was admitted to King Edward VII Hospital with complications related to her pregnancy. Two Australian radio announcers named Mel Greig and Michael Christian breached Catherine's medical privacy with a prank phone call to the hospital. Pretending to be Queen Elizabeth and Prince Charles, Greig and Christian asked questions about Catherines's condition. Jacintha Saldanha, a hospital nurse, fell for the prank and transferred the call to other nurses who released details to the duo.

After the radio broadcast, news stations all over the world reported what had happened, and the hospital instituted new rules to strengthen patient privacy protections. Although the hospital claimed that Saldanha was not disciplined for her actions, Saldanha, who had a history of mental disorders, committed suicide three days later. Her suicide note blamed the radio hosts for causing her death. Greig and Christian were widely criticized and were suspended from their jobs. Several months later, Christian reportedly went back to work in another capacity at the radio station, but Greig claimed that she was too traumatized to go back to work. As of July 2013, she had filed a lawsuit against her employer, blaming them for her actions and claiming that they failed to provide a safe workplace.

(doctors enrolled in postgraduate training). The manual contained instructions telling the doctors how to use a nonsecure Dropbox site to transfer patient records from their iPads to hospital computers. It also posted a user name and password for all the doctors to use on the site. After a cybersecurity expert discovered the manual online, the university removed it from the Internet.

Other security experts have cited this incident as an example of how doctors value the convenience of using mobile devices without thinking about how patient privacy may be affected. Some experts have warned that such inattention to security can result in dangers to entire computer networks, along with exposing patients to identity theft and other personal consequences. One scenario that a setup like the iPad-Dropbox could create is that hackers could plant "PDFs or other files that include harmful code that would be downloaded to all these iPads, and invade the hospital networks,"[36] states the technology website L'Atelier.

Patient data was also placed at risk in 2009–2010 when the managed health care company WellPoint carelessly allowed customers to apply for benefits using a nonsecure online form. This placed the EMRs of 612,402 people online for the world of Internet users to view. An OCR investigation concluded that WellPoint violated HIPAA rules and fined the company $1.7 million. HHS commented, "This case sends an important message to HIPAA-covered entities to take caution when implementing changes to their information systems, especially when these changes involve updates to Web-based applications."[37]

Social Media Breaches

Hospital employees have also violated patient privacy with online postings to their social media pages. In fact, the problem of employees posting photos and comments about patients on Facebook and other social media sites has become so prevalent at some hospitals that rules which prohibit employees from accessing these sites at work have been implemented. In one case, a sixty-year-old patient named William Wells was admitted to St. Mary Medical Center in Long Beach, California, after being stabbed numerous times. Instead of doing their jobs, several nurses and other employees took cell phone photos of Wells's gruesome injuries and posted the photos on Facebook. Most of the employees were fired.

Similar occurrences have been perpetrated by doctors. In 2010, for example, Alexandra Thran, an emergency room physician at Westerly Hospital in Rhode Island, posted details about several patients on Facebook. Although she did not post names, she was reprimanded and fined $500 because the details she posted allowed people in the community to identify the patients. Also in 2010, several doctors in

Australia were warned by a regional medical association to stop posting patient information on Facebook. One doctor in particular was criticized for making "flippant and derogatory" remarks. Michael Steiner of the Australian Medical Association stated that "doctors need to remember at all times the importance of patient confidentiality. I cannot believe that anyone would be silly enough to do this."[38]

In addition to getting hospital workers fired or disciplined, in several instances inappropriate postings have led to lawsuits. In June 2013, for example, surgeon Vinaya Puppala of Northwestern Memorial Hospital in Chicago took photos of an unconscious, intoxicated, former Northwestern University student named Elena Chernyakova. He posted the photos on Facebook and Instagram, along with comments about the situation. Puppala refused to delete the photos after hospital administrators asked him to do so, and Chernyakova later filed a $1.5 million lawsuit against Puppala and the hospital for violating her privacy. The lawsuit claims that Chernyakova had the "potential to someday work for Fortune 500 companies, which may now not occur because of said photographs."[39] The lawsuit has not yet been resolved in court.

In another case, anesthesiologist Patrick Yang decided to play a prank on a hospital employee, Veronica Valdez, while Valdez was undergoing surgery. Yang pasted stickers on Valdez's face to make it look like she had a moustache and pasted teardrop stickers under one eye. A nursing attendant took pictures with her cell phone and posted the photos on Facebook. Yang stated that he thought Valdez would laugh at the prank, but instead of being amused, Valdez said she felt humiliated enough to quit her job. She also filed a lawsuit against Yang and the hospital.

Deliberate Breaches

Many patient privacy breaches, unlike those involving careless or thoughtless online postings, are committed deliberately for some sort of personal gain by medical employees or outside hackers. Like Lawanda Jackson at UCLA Medical Center, some employees breach patient privacy so they can sell celebrity patient information to tabloids or noncelebrity patient information to identity thieves. In one major breach in 2012, a medical technician at Howard University was convicted of selling patients' medical and financial information for $500 to $800 per file to criminals who used the data to steal the patients' identities. The criminals posed as the patients to receive health care that was then billed to each patient's insurance company. Besides the financial and emotional devastation that this type of identity theft can cause, it also results in information about the criminals' medical conditions being entered into the real patients' charts. This leads to confusion and possibly to the wrong treatments being administered to patients. According to the World Privacy Forum, "Medical identity theft typically leaves a trail of falsified information in medical records that can plague victims' medical and financial lives for years."[40]

> "Medical identity theft typically leaves a trail of falsified information in medical records that can plague victims' medical and financial lives for years."[40]
>
> *—The World Privacy Forum.*

In another case involving the sale of medical data, Isis Machado, an office worker at the Cleveland Clinic in Florida, sold the EMRs of more than one thousand patients to her cousin, Fernando Ferrer, for five to ten dollars each. Ferrer used the information to submit $7 million worth of fraudulent charges to Medicare. Both Machado and Ferrer served time in prison and were forced to repay the stolen money.

Sometimes employees who snoop in patient records have motives other than money. In 2010, for example, surgeon Huping Zhou was convicted of HIPAA violations after he accessed the EMRs of coworkers and other patients in retaliation for being fired from his job. Zhou served four months in prison. In another case, Andrea Smith, a nurse in Arkansas, illegally accessed the EMRs of a patient who was involved in a lawsuit. Smith gave the records to her attorney husband, John, so he could use the information against the patient in court. Both Andrea and John Smith were convicted of violating HIPAA rules for personal gain and malicious harm.

Outside Hackers

In instances where outside hackers rather than medical employees access EMRs, the source of the resulting crimes is more difficult to track down because these hackers hide behind false online identities. Many hackers are also located overseas, which makes finding and prosecuting them almost impossible.

Foreign hackers often use the information they access in the EMRs to open credit card accounts in patients' names and then purchase huge amounts of goods and services with the credit cards. They also sell the information to others for similar purposes. In addition to committing these types of crimes, foreign hackers are now committing a relatively new type of crime known as medical data blackmail. This involves hackers holding computer data "hostage" and demanding ransom money to release the data, just like kidnappers often do when they abduct people. The first known case of medical data blackmail occurred in 2003 and involved Lubna Baloch. Since that time the number and sophistication of these crimes have increased, and an article in the technology publication *Fast Company* calls medical blackmail the "next frontier"[41] for computer hackers.

> "Based on the number of practices moving to electronic health records, many more of these types of breaches should be expected."[42]
>
> —*Journalist Jordan Robertson.*

In one recent occurrence, in December 2012, Russian hackers remotely took over the databases of the Miami Family Medical Center in Queensland, Australia, encrypted the files so they were useless unless "unlocked," and demanded a ransom of $4,000. The clinic had antivirus and anti-spyware programs in place, and no one figured out how the hackers gained access. The clinic, however, had been storing their data in backup files on a computer outside the office, so they were able to recover their files without paying the ransom.

Other victims of blackmail have also refused to pay. In 2008, for example, the prescription drug manager Express Scripts received a data ransom note and went to the police instead of paying. In 2012 the Surgeons of Lake County medical group in Illinois did the same thing. Some clinics and hospitals, however, have paid ransoms to regain use of their EMRs. After several instances of medical data blackmail in 2012, a Bloomberg News article stated, "Based on the number of practices moving to electronic health records, many more of these types of breaches should be expected."[42]

The Consequences of Breaches

Whether privacy breaches involve hacking, stealing computers, or posting data online, the consequences for affected patients can range from embarrassment to financial ruin, lost jobs, lost confidence in medical care, and worsening health problems. One instance where a privacy breach worsened an existing illness occurred in England in 2008, when a health care worker at Derriford Hospital accessed her

Hackers who breach medical record databases might seek patient names and other personal information. With this stolen data a hacker can, for instance, open fraudulent credit card accounts.

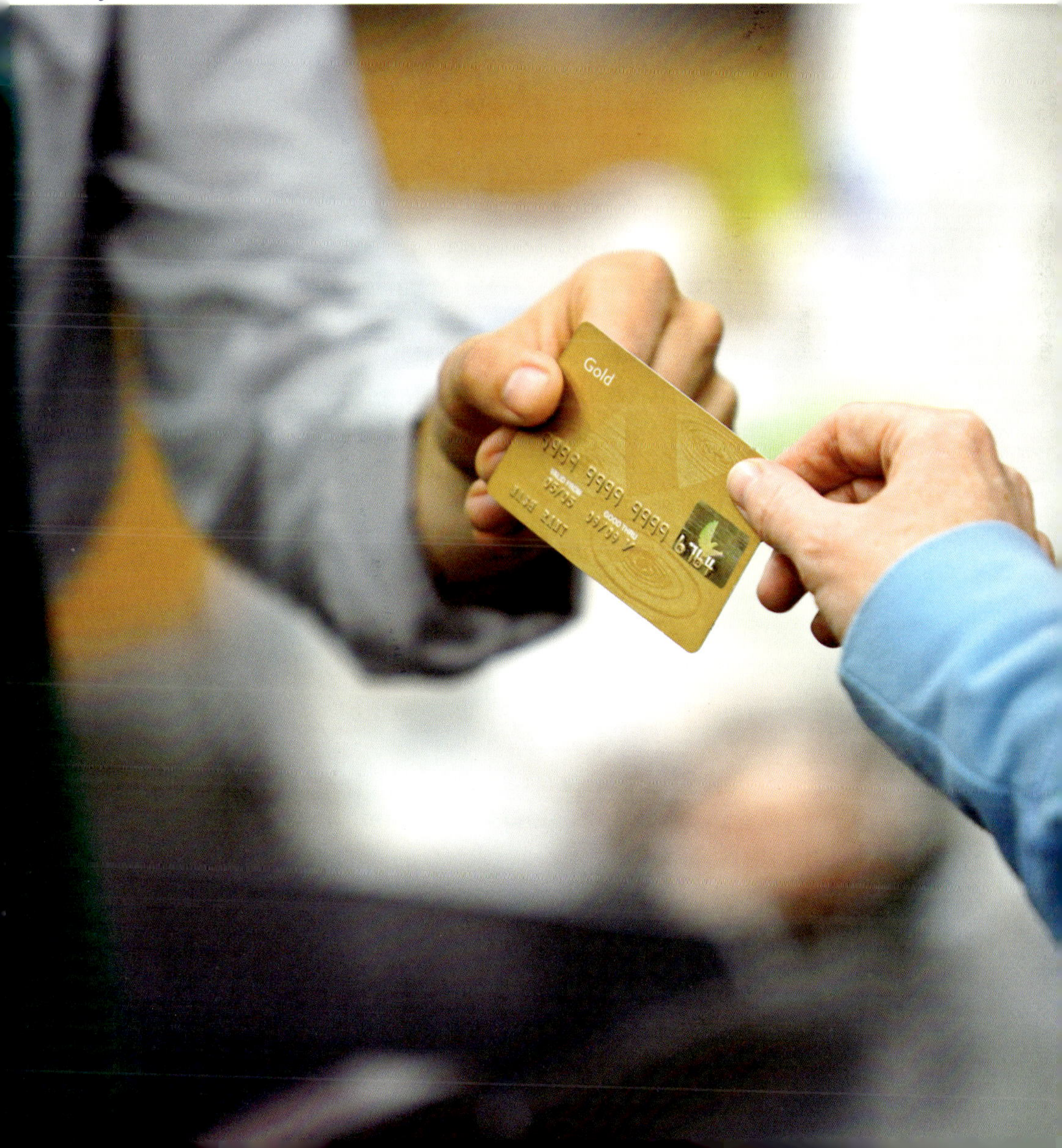

Antiabortion Activists and Patient Privacy

Antiabortion activists often breach patients' medical privacy to advance their own agenda. In one case, Daniel and Angela Michael, who routinely protested outside an abortion clinic in Illinois, photographed a woman who was rushed from the clinic to St. Elizabeth's Hospital after experiencing complications. The Michaels then fraudulently obtained the woman's medical records and posted the records and photo online.

In another case, a New York woman traveled to New Mexico to receive a late-term abortion. She suffered complications and was rushed to a hospital. Afterward, the antiabortion group Operation Rescue demanded an investigation by the state medical board because they knew the investigation would lead to the woman's medical records being released to attorneys and publicly debated in court.

Many similar cases have occurred. Antiabortion activists routinely photograph women and their cars' license plates as they enter abortion clinics, then post the photos online to try to shame the women. Some have posted women's photos and names on "hit lists" that encourage others to murder them.

Although these tactics violate medical privacy laws, authorities are reluctant to take action unless the activists make specific threats or physically assault women who choose to receive abortions. Some states have created "buffer zones" around abortion clinics that restrict intruders, but this has done little to curtail the privacy abuses. Antiabortion activists claim they are exercising their First Amendment rights to free speech, but privacy rights experts state that these rights do not extend to breaches of medical privacy.

ex-boyfriend's medical records and used the information to locate his family members. She then verbally harassed the ex-boyfriend, Sean Grinyer, in front of his family. Grinyer, who suffered from a mental disorder called paranoid personality disorder, claimed in a lawsuit that the woman's actions led him to experience a full-blown nervous breakdown. The courts ruled that the hospital had to pay him the British pound equivalent of about $25,000.

People with existing mental disorders are especially susceptible to experiencing severe emotional consequences from privacy breaches. After the Stanford University Hospital incident in which patient data was left online and unprotected for almost a year, one psychiatric patient's mother refrained from letting her son know about the breach because she was worried about his reaction. "My son, I can tell you, is fragile and confused enough that this would have sent him over the edge,"[43] she stated in a newspaper article.

The consequences of hospital database or medical record breaches can be even more severe than emotional harm. Even if these electronic databases are not posted online, hackers can use the Internet to break in to them and can insert computer viruses or other malware. Such an attack could easily shut down a hospital's entire computer network, causing critical computer-controlled medical devices such as ventilators and intravenous pumps to stop working. This could endanger many patients' lives. Even independently controlled electronic devices such as the insulin pumps, which many diabetics use every day, are susceptible to being hacked. If this happens the hackers can instruct the device to administer lethal doses of medication. Computer security expert Jay Radcliffe demonstrated how this could be done at a 2013 security conference.

At the same conference, another presentation showed that hackers could take over electronic pacemakers that are implanted in the chests of heart patients to control their heartbeats. A terrorist supposedly used this method to assassinate the vice president in an episode of the fictional television show *Homeland*. Although nothing like this has happened in real life, cybersecurity experts have warned that unless health care providers and medical device manufacturers improve their security systems, these and other threats to patient health will make the consequences of everyday breaches of EMRs seem insignificant.

Chapter 5

Health Care Privacy Enforcement and Effectiveness

Balancing patient privacy while promoting the free flow of information to improve health care is challenging, and new challenges emerge regularly as technology advances. In the United States, HHS and its OCR attempt to keep pace with these challenges through education and enforcement of HIPAA rules. HHS provides education programs to those who work in the health care field to ensure that everyone from doctors and nurses to office workers and technicians are aware of and practice patient privacy protection. Professional organizations and colleges that train and certify people in health information management also help meet the need for secure handling and protection of patient data.

Education on Mobile Devices

One area of technology that has spurred recent education programs is the use of wireless phones and computers to store and transmit health records. In December 2012 HHS launched the Mobile Devices: Know the RISKS. Take the STEPS. PROTECT and SECURE Health Information program that includes fact sheets, posters, and videos to teach health care providers the essentials. Joy Pritts of the Office of the National Coordinator for Health Information Technology emphasizes the importance of the program in a press release: "The use of mobile health technology holds great promise in improving health and health care, but the loss of health information can have a devastating impact on the trust patients have in their providers. It's important that these tools are used correctly."[44]

This program recommends many methods of improving mobile device security. For example, using strong passwords with upper- and lowercase letters and numbers makes it difficult for hackers to guess these passwords. The program also recommends that users activate locking features which shut down information being viewed after a set amount of time and that they install remote wiping and disabling capabilities to remotely erase data if the device is lost or stolen. Deleting file-sharing software, encrypting data, and using up-to-date firewalls and malware-blocking software are also important tips advocated by the HHS program.

Since mobile devices are responsible for many data breaches, the program basically strives to make users aware of the many ways in which they leave patient data vulnerable. This includes being careless about physically locking up mobile devices and leaving devices vulnerable to hacking and malware by using public Wi-Fi connections in cafes, airports, and other places.

> "The use of mobile health technology holds great promise in improving health and health care, but the loss of health information can have a devastating impact on the trust patients have in their providers."[44]
>
> —*Joy Pritts of the Office of the National Coordinator for Health Information Technology.*

HIPAA Enforcement

In addition to mandating HIPAA-related education and training programs for health care workers, HHS and OCR are responsible for investigating and enforcing HIPAA rules. The HIPAA Breach Notification Rule requires providers to notify OCR about any data breaches that affect five hundred or more people. Many times providers report breaches that involve fewer numbers as well. OCR then investigates and may prosecute these offenses in federal court.

The HITECH Act of 2009 grants state attorneys general the right to investigate and prosecute HIPAA violations in state courts as well. Attorneys general are the chief legal advisers and prosecutors in each state. Like OCR, these state-based enforcers can impose fines, jail sentences, and other sanctions for HIPAA breaches. Most state and federal penalties include mandatory employee retraining and specific

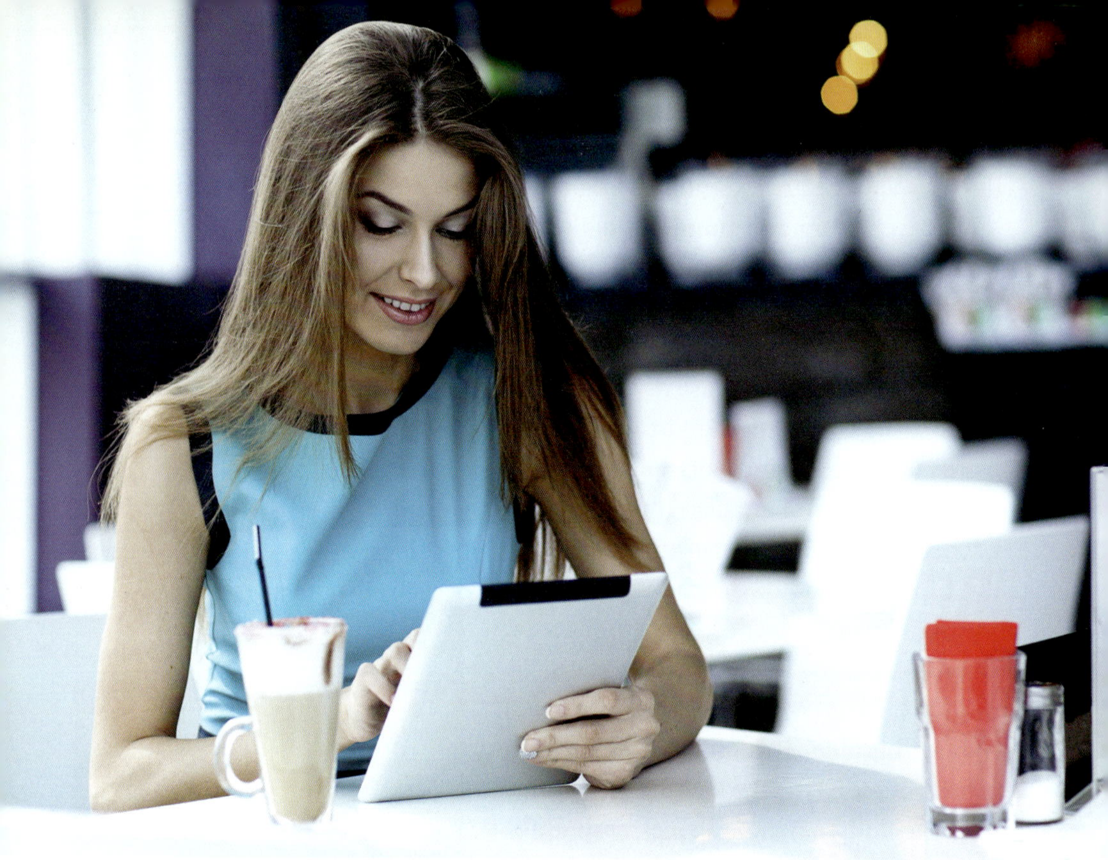

Mobile devices such as tablets and laptops are often involved in medical data breaches. To reduce this vulnerability, users are encouraged to lock up these devices when they are not in use for their designated purpose.

security policy changes, depending on the reasons for the breach. In May 2013, for example, Idaho State University's Pocatello Family Medicine Clinic paid a $400,000 fine and was directed to install and maintain adequate firewall protections on their computers. The clinic left the EMRs of 17,500 patients vulnerable after information technology managers disabled their computer firewalls so patient EMRs could be easily shared throughout the university network.

In another case, a health maintenance organization (HMO) did not obtain a patient's signature on a HIPAA form before releasing the patient's EMRs to a disability insurance company. OCR required the HMO to create HIPAA-compliant forms and to train employees to release information only if a signed form was in a patient's file. As a result of these types of enforcement activities, many health care providers have improved their procedures. As HHS states, "The corrective actions obtained by OCR from covered entities have resulted in systemic change that has improved the privacy protection of health information for all individuals they serve."[45]

Despite such positive developments, however, a 2012 study by the Ponemon Institute revealed that the number of EMR breaches has increased since 2010. Most of the increases are attributed to the use of mobile devices, file-sharing applications, employee mistakes, hackers, and careless practices by business associates of covered entities. Ninety-four percent of health care organizations reported having at least one data breach between 2010 and 2012, and 45 percent reported having more than five breaches. Two-thirds of these health organizations reported that they do not have adequate methods of detecting the medical identity theft that often results from these breaches, and less than half conduct annual privacy and security risk assessments.

"The corrective actions obtained by OCR from covered entities have resulted in systemic change that has improved the privacy protection of health information for all individuals they serve."[45]

—US Department of Health and Human Services.

Is HIPAA Effective?

These types of statistics have led many health organizations and privacy advocates to question HIPAA's effectiveness. The Institute of Medicine, for instance, states in a report that HIPAA "does not protect privacy as well as it should."[46] Some privacy advocates believe that besides being ineffective, HIPAA is not designed to actually protect patient privacy. In an article on the Western Center for Journalism website, author Doug Book writes:

> Few people realize that the HIPAA "privacy" form shoved under the nose of every individual visiting a hospital or doctor's office has NOTHING whatever to do with the preservation of patient privacy. Nor does it mean that patient consent will be required before a healthcare provider may share their records. On the contrary, signing the form simply means the patient has been advised that his most private medical (and other) information may be legally accessed by some 2.2 million entities, many having nothing to do with either health or treatment.[47]

Book is referring to the many business associates of covered entities and the government in his calculation of the number of individuals and organizations that have access to patient records. Indeed, one aspect of HIPAA that many people resent is that so many people who have no role in patient care are allowed access to EMRs without the knowledge or approval of patients. One man whose records were inappropriately accessed states in a *Los Angeles Times* article, "I don't think anything is secure anymore. It's nobody's business unless I choose it to be someone's business."[48]

> "Few people realize that the HIPAA 'privacy' form shoved under the nose of every individual visiting a hospital or doctor's office has NOTHING whatever to do with the preservation of patient privacy."[47]
>
> —*Author Doug Book.*

Many people also resent the fact that HIPAA allows health care providers to sell patients' medical information without permission. While HIPAA mandates that most of this information must have identifying data removed, privacy experts have demonstrated that this "de-identified" data can be easily identified. For example, Latanya Sweeny, director of the Data Privacy Lab at Harvard University, created a computer program that cross-references states' medical data with news reports and public records. Sweeny then purchased "de-identified" hospital records from a Washington health department and used the program to correctly identify thirty-five patients.

For these reasons, many privacy advocates have demanded that HIPAA be changed to limit the sale of patient records and the ability of anyone outside the health care field to access these records. In January 2013 HHS responded to such concerns by amending HIPAA to increase penalties for violations and require health care providers and their business associates to implement stricter privacy and security measures. The change also limits the sale of patient information without the patient's permission. "The new rule will help protect patient privacy and safeguard patient health information in an ever-expanding digital age,"[49] states HHS secretary Kathleen Sebelius in a press release.

Health Information Management

Widespread concerns about electronic health information privacy have led to a demand for professionals who are specially trained in health information management. People can train to properly handle and protect electronic medical records in colleges and through health information management organizations that offer education and career training programs. These organizations also grant degrees and certifications in health information management to qualified individuals. For example, the American Health Information Management Association (AHIMA) is one professional organization that educates, certifies, and advocates for health information management professionals.

Health information managers work in doctor's offices, hospitals, nursing homes, pharmacies, information technology firms, insurance companies, and other industries. According to AHIMA, "Having skilled HIM [health information management] professionals on staff insures an organization has the right information on hand when and where it is needed while maintaining the highest standards of data integrity, confidentiality, and security."

American Health Information Management Association, "AHIMA Facts." www.ahima.org.

Other Consequences of HIPAA

While health care providers agree that protecting patient privacy is important, many also believe that HIPAA goes overboard in regulating and enforcing patient privacy. In many instances, fear of being penalized by OCR has led providers to go to somewhat ridiculous lengths to ensure that they are complying with the law. For instance, being a HIPAA-covered entity forced all departments, including the library, at the Johns Hopkins University Hospital to conform to HIPAA rules. The Johns Hopkins hospital medical library contains the Chesney Medical Archives, which include original books, letters, and other documents relating to the history of the hospital and the schools of medicine, nursing, and public health. These documents are available to students and outside scholars for reference purposes. Because of HIPAA, the archive staff had to spend thousands of hours reading through thousands of documents to delete anything that revealed personal health information. For example, one nineteenth-century document mentioned that a particular doctor died of cancer. The doctor's name had to be removed from the document because he could not grant permission (since he was dead) for this information to be viewed by the public. Had the same document been housed at a historical society or public library rather than at a hospital library, no such editing would have been necessary because HIPAA does not apply to these places.

"What most people care most about is not simply *restricting* the flow of information, but ensuring that it flows *appropriately*."[51]

—Legal and technology expert Helen Nissenbaum.

Institutions that conduct medical research have also claimed that complying with the HIPAA privacy rules hinders their research and also sometimes conflicts with other laws that govern this type of research. Research centers must often hire additional staff members just to monitor and submit paperwork on HIPAA compliance. Researchers themselves must devote a great deal of time to filling out and explaining HIPAA paperwork to patients enrolled in research studies. The privacy forms are so numerous and complicated, researchers report, that many patients are intimidated and refuse to participate in important clinical research. Many medical research advocates have therefore urged lawmakers to exempt research from HIPAA rules. According to the authors of an Association of Academic Health Centers report, "Research was not intended to be governed by the HIPAA Privacy Rule, but neither was it exempted from the regulation."[50]

Balancing Technology and Privacy

The perception that HIPAA impedes research and fails to adequately protect patient privacy has contributed to ongoing demands for changing or even replacing the law. Some medical and legal experts have also proposed that the HIPAA and HITECH initiatives to increase the use of EMRs should be halted, but most believe that EMRs have advantages and should be encouraged. A 2012 survey, for example, revealed that more than 70 percent of the physicians that have implemented EMRs are pleased with the convenience of being able to access patient records wherever they are and believe that EMRs can enhance patient care.

About 70 percent of doctors who have switched from paper to electronic records find that electronic records enhance patient care. Nevertheless, most health professionals, consumers, and policy makers believe that privacy protections for such records must be strengthened.

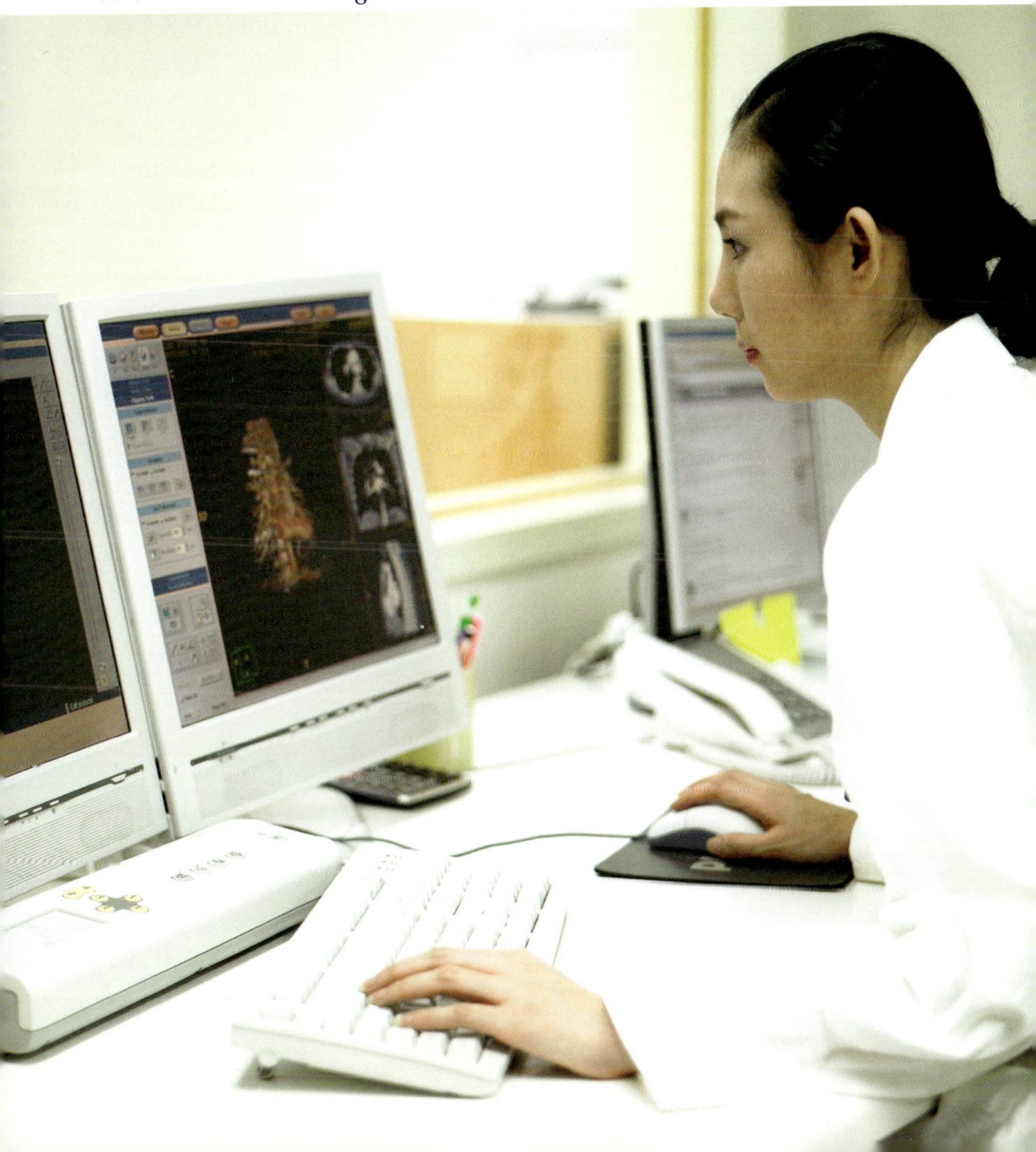

Medical Privacy and Gun Control

Issues of medical privacy have emerged in ongoing efforts to reduce gun violence in the United States. Federal and state laws prohibit convicted criminals and severely mentally ill people from buying or owning guns. The FBI launched the National Instant Criminal Background Check System (NICS) in 1998 to allow gun sellers to run background checks on anyone trying to purchase a gun. However, because of HIPAA, state health departments have been reluctant to furnish the names of severely mentally ill people to NICS. Many with mental illnesses have therefore passed background checks.

In February 2013 HHS proposed an amendment to HIPAA that would remove barriers to reporting mental health data to NICS. This proposal is part of a new government plan to reduce gun violence after numerous mass shootings in the United States, such as the movie theater shooting in Colorado and the school shooting in Newtown, Connecticut. Most of the shooters in these cases had a history of mental illness.

Several mental health advocacy and privacy groups have expressed opposition to the proposed HIPAA changes. The National Association of State Mental Health Programs, for instance, writes in a letter to HHS that the amendment would "exacerbate the stigma faced by people with mental illnesses" and might discourage these individuals from seeking mental health treatment. However, a Pew Research Center survey found that 80 percent of Americans support efforts to prevent the mentally ill from buying guns and believe that sacrificing some privacy for public safety is warranted.

Quoted in iHealth Beat, "Groups Oppose HIPAA Changes for Gun-Purchase Database," June 13, 2013. www.ihealthbeat.org.

While many health care experts and patients agree that EMRs have advantages and are here to stay, all are equally insistent that patient privacy should be enhanced, either by overhauling or replacing HIPAA. Many patients and health care experts also believe that any HIPAA changes or new health care privacy laws should give patients more control over who may access their records. Legal and technology expert Helen Nissenbaum, for instance, writes in her book *Privacy in Context*, "What most people care most about is not simply *restricting* the flow of information, but ensuring that it flows *appropriately*."[51]

Deborah C. Peel builds on this viewpoint in a 2010 *Wall Street Journal* article, stating, "There is no need to choose between the benefits of technology and our rights to health privacy. Technologies already exist that enable each person to choose what information he is willing to share and what must remain private. Consent must be built into electronic systems up front so we can each choose the levels of privacy and sharing we prefer."[52]

Many privacy advocates agree with Peel's ideas, which essentially state that individuals, rather than the government and health care providers, should have the power to decide with whom their private medical information is shared. The Patient Privacy Rights organization, for example, has proposed eliminating the HIPAA consent forms which give health care providers the authority to share patient data with other doctors, insurance companies, or others involved in patient health care. Instead, patients would sign forms to express their wishes: "Informed consents should be direct 'one-to-one' consents, with a specific purpose and time frame. Those who are granted access should be clearly named or described."[53]

> "Consent must be built into electronic systems up front so we can each choose the levels of privacy and sharing we prefer."[52]
>
> —*Psychiatrist Deborah C. Peel.*

Steps Toward Patient Control

A 2012 study conducted by researchers at Clemson University found that most patients are in favor of this type of consent and control over their medical records. The study also found that most patients are willing to share some or all of their records with doctors other than their primary care doctor, but that very few (0 to 5 percent) are willing to give the government access to any of their health information.

While the January 2013 HIPAA Final Rule changes did not specifically address patient concerns about government access to their health information, these changes did heed patient desires to have more control. An HHS press release states that "The changes in the final rulemaking provide the public with increased protections and control of personal health information."[54] For example, the new rule prohibits health care providers from selling patient information without the patient's permission. It also limits the ways in which marketers can use this information.

Patient control is also enhanced by provisions that allow people to ask for electronic copies of their records. These provisions also require health care providers to furnish these copies. Patients may also instruct their doctors to refrain from disclosing certain parts of their records to insurance companies if the patient has paid for specific services in cash. Under the new rule, doctors must agree to honor such requests in most cases.

Further changes give parents more control over how they can instruct health care providers to share information about a child's immunization records with schools when this is required by law. Previously, parents were required to issue such instructions in writing. Under the new rule, they have a choice of conveying these directions orally, by e-mail, or in writing. The Final Rule states that "We believe that the option to provide oral agreement for the disclosure of student immunization records will relieve burden on parents, schools, and covered entities while still giving parents the opportunity to consider whether to agree to the disclosure of this information."[55]

A New Era of Patient Engagement

The HIPAA changes do not give patients the complete control over their health information that many privacy advocates envision, but they do signal a new era of patient engagement and empowerment with regard to their health care privacy. Some countries have already shifted complete control over EMRs to patients. The Netherlands, for instance, is using a system where only the person who "owns" the data is allowed to share it. England and Canada are currently exploring similar systems. In the United States, the Department of Veterans Affairs (VA) is testing software technology that allows patients to control access to their records by logging onto the VA hospital website and filling out simple and specific consent forms.

Other types of patient control over EMRs have been proposed as well. A team of Microsoft researchers, for example, has proposed a system called Patient Controlled Encryption. This system gives patients the keys to encrypt various parts of their EMRs so certain health care providers or billing services do not have access to the encrypted sections. Another type of consent technology being explored is health record banks. Here, each time a patient receives health care, the new records are deposited in his or her personal online health bank account. These accounts have security features similar to those of banks that deal with money. Each patient decides when and how any health information can be withdrawn. Currently, several communities in Washington, Kentucky, Missouri, and Florida are developing such banks.

Whether any of the proposals to strengthen individuals' control over their health care privacy will be widely adopted in the United States remains to be seen. In the meantime, protecting patient privacy in the online world continues to challenge every person and institution involved in health care. Attorney Jim Pyles sums up the challenges in a *Bloomberg Businessweek* article: "Electronic health information is like nuclear energy. If it's harnessed and kept under tight control, it has potential for good. But if it gets out of control, the damage is incalculable."[56]

Source Notes

Introduction: Threats to Health Care Privacy

1. Quoted in Charles Ornstein, "Just 'Nosy,' Says Figure in Medical Data Scandal," *Los Angeles Times*, April 9, 2008. http://articles.latimes.com.
2. Sharyl J. Nass, Laura A. Levitt, and Lawrence O. Gostin, eds., *Beyond the HIPAA Privacy Rule: Enhancing Privacy, Improving Health Through Research*, Institute of Medicine and National Research Council. Washington, DC: National Academies Press, 2009, p. 77.
3. Quoted in Robert O'Harrow Jr., "Health-Care Sector Vulnerable to Hackers, Researchers Say," *Washington Post*, December 25, 2012. http://articles.washingtonpost.com.
4. Diane Black and Patrick Meehan, "Obamacare Poses Security Threat: Column," *USA Today*, August 21, 2013. www.usatoday.com.

Chapter 1: The Importance of Privacy

5. Judith Wagner DeCew, "Connecting Informational, 4th Amendment and Constitutional Privacy," Information Ethics and Policy Conference, University of Washington, April 25–26, 2013. http://infoethics.ischool.uw.edu.
6. John Locke, *The Second Treatise of Civil Government*, chap. 7, section 87, 1690. http://oregonstate.edu/instruct/phl302/texts/locke/locke2/locke2nd-a.html.
7. Locke, *The Second Treatise of Civil Government*, chap. 5, section 27. http://oregonstate.edu/instruct/phl302/texts/locke/locke2/locke2nd-a.html.
8. Daniel J. Solove, *Understanding Privacy*. Cambridge, MA: Harvard University Press, 2008, p. 33.
9. United Nations, "The Universal Declaration of Human Rights," December 10, 1948. www.un.org.

10. Samuel Warren and Louis Brandeis, "The Right to Privacy," *Harvard Law Review*, vol. 4, no. 5, December 15, 1890.
11. Charles A. Shoniregun, Kudakwashe Dube, and Fredrick Mtenzi, *Electronic Healthcare Information Security*. New York: Springer Science + Business Media, 2010, p. 2.
12. National Library of Medicine, "The Hippocratic Oath." www.nlm.nih.gov.
13. American Medical Association, "Patient Confidentiality." www.ama-assn.org.
14. Luke Davis et al. "Attitudes of First-Year Medical Students Toward the Confidentiality of Computerized Patient Records," *Journal of the American Medical Informatics Association*, January/February 1999, p. 54.

Chapter 2: Who Has Access to Private Medical Information?

15. American Medical Association, "HIPAA Security Rule: Frequently Asked Questions Regarding Encryption of Personal Health Information." www.ama-assn.org.
16. Bernhard Warner, "Doctors Like Electronic Medical Records, as Long as Patients Can't Touch Them," *Bloomberg Businessweek*, March 13, 2013. www.businessweek.com.
17. Privacy Rights Clearinghouse, "Fact Sheet 8: Medical Records Privacy." www.privacyrights.org.
18. US Department of Health and Human Services, "Standards for Privacy of Individually Identifiable Health Information." http://aspe.hhs.gov.
19. National Institute of Standards and Technology, "Safeguarding Health Information: Building Assurance Through HIPAA Security—2013." www.nist.gov.
20. Nass, Levitt, and Gostin, *Beyond the HIPAA Privacy Rule*, p. 1.
21. Quoted in Sonia Gupta, "The Hippocratic Oath and HIV: A Conflict of Ethics," *Yale Journal of Medicine and Law*, October 5, 2010. www.yalemedlaw.com.
22. American Health Information Management Association, "The Privacy and Security of Occupational Health Records." http://library.ahima.org.

23. US Department of Health and Human Services, "Does the HIPAA Privacy Rule Permit a Doctor to Discuss a Patient's Health Status, Treatment or Payment Arrangements with the Patient's Family and Friends?," www.hhs.gov.

Chapter 3: The Push for Electronic Medical Records

24. Stephan Kudyba, ed., *Healthcare Informatics*. Boca Raton, FL: CRC, 2010, p. 6.
25. Steve Denning, "Why Is Your Doctor Typing? Electronic Medical Records Run Amok," *Forbes*, April 25, 2013. www.forbes.com.
26. Quoted in HealthIT.gov, "Dr. Michael Gilbert and the Benefits of Electronic Health Records with Patients and Beyond," www.healthit.gov.
27. Quoted in National Public Radio, "Electronic Medical Records May Boost Patient Safety," July 15, 2013. www.npr.org.
28. Institute of Medicine, *Health IT and Patient Safety: Building Safer Systems for Better Care*. Washington, DC: National Academies Press, 2012, p. 1.
29. America's Watchtower, "Obamacare Privacy Intrusion Will Dwarf the NSA Spying Scandal," July 20, 2013. http://americaswatchtower.com.
30. Stacy Cowly, "How Obamacare's 'Privacy Nightmare' Database Really Works," CNN, July 24, 2013. http://money.cnn.com.
31. Joe Klein, "Sanity on Obamacare," *Time*, October 27, 2013. http://swampland.time.com.
32. Center for Democracy & Technology, "FAQ: HIPAA and 'Cloud Computing,'" August 7, 2013. www.cdt.org.
33. Christina Zarcadoolas et al. "Consumers' Perceptions of Patient-Accessible Electronic Medical Records," *Journal of Medical Internet Research* , August 2013. www.ncbi.nlm.nih.gov.

Chapter 4: Health Care Privacy Breaches and Their Effects

34. Quoted in Robert O'Harrow, "Health-Care Sector Vulnerable to Hackers, Researchers Say," *Washington Post*, December 25, 2012. http://articles.washingtonpost.com.

35. Kevin Sack, "Patient Data Posted Online in Major Breach of Privacy," *New York Times*, September 8, 2011. www.nytimes.com.
36. L'Atelier, "The Newly Digitized Healthcare Industry Is Vulnerable to Hacking," January 2, 2013. www.atelier.net.
37. US Department of Health and Human Services, "WellPoint Pays HHS $1.7 Million for Leaving Information Accessible over Internet." www.hhs.gov.
38. Quoted in Helen Pow, "Doctors Caught Revealing Secret Patient Information in Facebook Posts," *Sunday Telegraph* (Australia), September 25, 2010. www.news.com.au.
39. Quoted in Alana Abramson, "Chicago Doctor Accused of Posting Photos of Intoxicated Patient," ABC News, August 20, 2013. http://abcnews.go.com.
40. World Privacy Forum, "The Medical Identity Theft Information Page." www.worldprivacyforum.org.
41. Neal Ungerleider, "Medical Cybercrime: The Next Frontier," *Fast Company*. www.fastcompany.com.
42. Jordan Robertson, "Hackers Encrypt Health Records and Hold Data for Ransom," Bloomberg News, August 10, 2012. www.bloomberg.com.
43. Quoted in Sack, "Patient Data Posted Online in Major Breach of Privacy."

Chapter 5: Health Care Privacy Enforcement and Effectiveness

44. Quoted in US Department of Health and Human Services, "New Tools to Help Providers Protect Patient Data in Mobile Devices," December 12, 2012. www.hhs.gov.
45. US Department of Health and Human Services, "HIPAA Enforcement; Health Information Privacy." www.hhs.gov.
46. Nass, Levitt, and Gostin, eds., *Beyond the HIPAA Privacy Rule*, p. 2.
47. Doug Book, "Healthcare Privacy Law Guarantees Anything BUT Privacy," Western Center for Journalism. www.westernjournalism.com.
48. Quoted in *Los Angeles Times*, "Hacker Targets Files at Medical Center," December 11, 2000. http://articles.latimes.com.

49. Quoted in US Department of Health and Human Services, "New Rule Protects Patient Privacy, Secures Health Information," January 17, 2013. www.hhs.gov.
50. Mindy J. Steinberg and Elaine R. Rubin, "The HIPAA Privacy Rule: Lacks Patient Benefit, Impedes Research Growth," Association of Academic Health Centers. www.aahcdc.org.
51. Helen Nissenbaum, *Privacy in Context*. Stanford, CA: Stanford Law Books, 2010, p. 1.
52. Deborah C. Peel, "Your Medical Records Aren't Secure," *Wall Street Journal*, March 23, 2010. http://online.wsj.com.
53. Patient Privacy Rights, "The Case for Informed Consent," August 2010. http://patientprivacyrights.org.
54. US Department of Health and Human Services, "New Rule Protects Patient Privacy, Secures Health Information," press release, January 17, 2013.
55. *Federal Register*, "Modifications to the HIPAA Privacy, Security, Enforcement, and Breach Notification Rules Under the Health Information Technology for Economic and Clinical Health Act and the Genetic Information Nondiscrimination Act; Other Modifications to the HIPAA Rules." www.federalregister.gov.
56. Quoted in *Bloomberg Businessweek*, "Your Not-So-Secret Medical History," August 12, 2013, p. 42.

Online Privacy Tips

Basic Security

- Use security software to block viruses and malware. Keep it up to date.
- Use passwords at least eight characters long. Add numerals and punctuation to make them harder to guess.
- Back up important data to a flash or USB drive or an online service.

E-mail and Messaging

- Do not click on web links or attachments in e-mail or text messages unless you are expecting them. (Strange messages from a friend may indicate that their account has been "hijacked.")
- Beware of "scary" messages that claim to be from a bank or government agency. Contact the agency directly if you think there might be a problem.
- Do not put credit card numbers or other sensitive information in e-mail or text messages.

Web and Social Networks

- Learn about browser features that can enhance security and privacy.
- Find and use the privacy settings for Facebook, Twitter, and other social networks.
- Do not post personal details or other information that you wouldn't want a stranger to know.

Banking and E-Commerce

- Make payments only on secure web pages (indicated by https:// in the address and a padlock symbol).

- Do not do banking or make online purchases on a public Wifi network.
- Monitor bank and credit card accounts regularly for signs of fraud.

Mobile Devices

- Protect your phone or tablet with a passcode.
- Install software that allows you to track or disable lost or stolen devices.
- Install apps from only trusted sources.
- Check settings to see what information apps may be obtaining from your device.

Finally . . .

- Think before you hit "Send." You cannot take your words back.
- Common sense and courtesy can go a long way.

Related Organizations and Websites

American Health Information Management Association (AHIMA)

233 N. Michigan Ave., 21st Floor
Chicago, IL 60601
phone: (312) 233-1100
website: www.ahima.org

AHIMA is an organization that advocates for and certifies health information managers. Its website contains information on health care privacy issues.

American Medical Association (AMA)

AMA Plaza
330 N. Wabash Ave.
Chicago, IL 60611-5885
phone: (800) 621-8335
website: www.ama-assn.org

The American Medical Association is a professional organization for doctors that offers numerous articles on privacy issues on its website.

Center for Democracy and Technology

16341 I St. NW, #1100
Washington, DC 20006
phone: (202) 637-9800
website: www.cdt.org

The Center for Democracy and Technology is a nonprofit organization that advocates for free speech rights on the Internet. Its Health Privacy Project addresses health privacy issues related to the Internet.

Citizens' Council for Health Freedom

161 St. Anthony Ave., Suite 923
St. Paul, MN 55103
phone: (651) 646-8935
website: www.cchfreedom.org

The Citizens' Council for Health Freedom is a nonprofit organization that advocates for the rights of Americans to make health care decisions and to maintain doctor-patient confidentiality that is free from government intrusion.

Electronic Privacy Information Center

1718 Connecticut Ave. NW, Suite 200
Washington, DC 20009
phone: (202) 483-1140
website: http://epic.org

The Electronic Privacy Information Center is a public interest research center that publishes reports and books about privacy in the online world.

Office for Civil Rights

US Department of Health and Human Services
200 Independence Ave. SW, Room 509F
Washington, DC 20201
phone: (800) 368-1019
website: www.hhs.gov

The Office for Civil Rights enforces provisions of the health care privacy laws in the United States. Its website provides information on enforcement activities and cases.

Office of the National Coordinator for Health Information Technology

US Department of Health and Human Services
200 Independence Ave. SW, Suite 729-D
Washington, DC 20201
phone: (202) 690-7151
website: www.healthit.gov

The National Coordinator for Health Information Technology is part of the Department of Health and Human Services that informs the public about health information technology and develops standards that coordinate national and state health information technology regulations.

Patient Privacy Rights

1006 Mopac Circle, Suite 102
Austin, TX 78746
phone: (512) 732-0033
website: http://patientprivacyrights.org

Patient Privacy Rights is a nonprofit organization that works to support the health privacy of Americans. Its website offers information on health care privacy issues.

Privacy Rights Clearinghouse

3108 Fifth Ave., Suite A
San Diego, CA 92103
phone: (619) 298-3396
website: www.privacyrights.org

The Privacy Rights Clearinghouse is a nonprofit organization that educates and empowers individuals about their privacy rights. Its website contains information about health care privacy issues.

For Further Research

Books

Stephen Currie, *How Is the Internet Eroding Privacy Rights?* San Diego, CA: ReferencePoint, 2014.

Gale, ed., *Teens and Privacy*. Farmington Hills, MI: Greenhaven, 2011.

Jacqueline Klosek, *Protecting Your Health Privacy: A Citizen's Guide to Safeguarding the Security of Your Medical Information*. Santa Barbara, CA: Praeger, 2010.

Betsy Kuhn, *Prying Eyes: Privacy in the Twenty-First Century*. Minneapolis, MN: Twenty-First Century, 2008.

Noel Merino, ed., *Privacy*. Farmington Hills, MI: Greenhaven, 2012.

Daniel J. Solove, *Understanding Privacy*. Cambridge, MA: Harvard University Press, 2008.

Internet Sources

National Public Radio, "Electronic Medical Records May Boost Patient Safety," July 15, 2013. www.npr.org/templates/story/story.php?storyId=202401672.

The Office of the National Coordinator for Health Information Technology, "Health IT: Advancing America's Health Care." www.healthit.gov/sites/default/files/pdf/health-information-technology-fact-sheet.pdf.

The Office of the National Coordinator for Health Information Technology, "Protecting Your Privacy and Security." www.healthit.gov/sites/default/files/pdf/health-information-privacy-and-security.pdf.

Helen Pow, "Doctors Caught Revealing Secret Patient Information in Facebook Posts," (Australia) *Sunday Telegraph*, September 25, 2010. www.news.com.au/technology/doctors-caught-revealing-secret-information-on-facebook/story-e6frfrnr-1225929424789.

Teens Health from Nemours, "Your Medical Records." http://kidshealth.org/teen/your_body/health_basics/medical_records.html.

Michael Tennant, "Say Goodbye to Medical Privacy Under ObamaCare," *New American*, June 17, 2013. http://thenewamerican.com/usnews/health-care/item/15738-say-goodbye-to-medical-privacy-under-obamacare.

Eric Whitney, "Doctors Heed Prescription for Computerized Records," National Public Radio, July 15, 2013. www.npr.org/blogs/health/2013/07/15/201410052/doctors-take-prescription-for-computerized-records.

Index